Get Through

MRCPsych Part 2:
Clinical Exam: Long Case Presentations

This book is dedicated to:

My beloved wife Dr Mythili Varadan, my beloved sister Mrs Sri Vidhya Rajasekharan and to my respected teachers of psychiatry: Dr Rajaram Mohan, Dr Priscilla Read and Dr Rhinedd Toms

Get Through
MRCPsych Part 2: Clinical Exam: Long Case Presentations

Sree Prathap Mohana Murthy MB BS MRCPsych
South West London and St. George's Mental Health NHS Trust, London

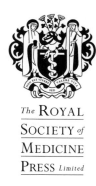

The ROYAL
SOCIETY of
MEDICINE
PRESS Limited

© 2006 Royal Society of Medicine Press Ltd
Published by the Royal Society of Medicine Press Ltd
1 Wimpole Street, London W1G 0AE, UK
Tel: +44 (0)20 7290 2921
Fax: +44 (0)20 7290 2929
Email: publishing@rsm.ac.uk
Website: www.rsmpress.co.uk

British Library Cataloguing in Publication Data
A catalogue record for this book is available from the British Library

ISBN 1-85315-684-1

Distribution in Europe and Rest of World:
Marston Book Services Ltd
PO Box 269 Abingdon Oxon OX14 4YN, UK Tel: +44 (0)1235 465500
Fax: +44 (0)1235 465555
Email: direct.order@marston.co.uk

Distribution in the USA and Canada:
Royal Society of Medicine Press Ltd
c/o BookMasters Inc
30 Amberwood Parkway
Ashland, OH 44805, USA
Tel: +1 800 247 6553/ +1 800 266 5564
Fax: +1 419 281 6883
Email: order@bookmasters.com

Distribution in Australia and New Zealand:
Elsevier Australia 30-52 Smidmore Street Marrikville NSW 2204, Australia
Tel: +61 2 9517 8999
Fax: +61 2 9517 2249
Email: service@elsevier.com.au

Typeset by Phoenix Photosetting, Chatham, Kent
Printed in the UK by Bell & Bain Ltd, Glasgow

Contents

Preface

The MRCPsych part 2 clinical examination consists of two main parts: 1) individual patient assessment and 2) a structured oral examination (SOE), also called patient management problems (PMPs).

The individual patient assessment is now the only full clinical exam and focuses on the following tasks:

- History (presenting the history)
- Mental state examination
- Physical examination
- Discussing the possible differential diagnosis
- Examination in front of the examiners (observed interview tasks)
- Aetiological formulation
- Investigations
- Management
- Prognosis-review of the possible outcomes.

Each candidate will have 1 hour to examine a patient and to organize their thoughts before an interview with the examiners that is scheduled to occupy 30 minutes.

The discussion with the examiners will cover the following topics:

- *Assessment* (approximately 10 minutes): This involves outlining the salient features in the history and the relevant findings on the mental state examination, the physical examination, the diagnosis and the differential diagnosis
- *Interview with the patient* (approximately 10 minutes): You will be asked to interview the patient in one or two areas from the history or examination of the mental state in front of the examiners
- *Management* (approximately 10 minutes): This involves further detailed integration of investigations, short-term and long-term management (biopsychosocial model and multidisciplinary approach is expected), aetiological formulation and prognosis, which involves review of the possible outcomes.

The examiners may also raise general clinical or specific questions relevant to the particular case.

This is an essential revision tool for all candidates preparing for the MRCPsych part 2 clinical examination. It highlights the areas that should be focused on to pass the long case presentation, and each task is discussed in detail in the relevant chapters.

This book will not only prepare you for the examination but will also help you to face the clinical situations confidently and effectively.

The answers that I have given should be used as a guide to form your own responses. However, reference to standard textbooks is also recommended.

Good luck.
Sree Prathap

1

History taking and mental state examination

How to take a history

- The history taking should begin with a courteous introduction and explanation of the interview, and any patient questions and concerns should be addressed
- Don't be hurried; act naturally, and be genuine, polite and professional with the patient
- Be respectful and empathetic with the patient
- Do not disagree with improbable assertions, such as delusional ideas or other psychotic phenomena, but avoid debating them
- Do not focus too much on irrelevancies, but try to redirect the flow of conversation and tailor the interview accordingly
- Keep safety issues in mind throughout the assessment
- The closure of the interview should be generally supportive and should include thanks and provide an opportunity for the patient to ask questions or add any other information that is significant to the case
- There are different schools of thought regarding the subheadings of a history, but the following format is usually accepted by most examiners:

    Demographic details
    Reason for referral
    Chief complaints
    History of presenting compliants
    Screening questions: direct questioning
    Past psychiatric history
    Past medical history
    Current medications
    Family history

Personal history
Current social circumstances
Drug and alcohol history
Forensic history
Premorbid personality
Mental state examination
- Lastly, tell a plain story plainly.

Demographic data

- Name
- Age
- Sex
- Marital status
- Employment status
- Occupation
- Date of admission
- Legal status.

Reason for referral

- How did you come into the hospital?
- Who referred you?
- When were you referred?
- Why were you referred?
- Did you come of your own free will or were you forced to come?

Chief complaints

Establish exactly why the patient came to see the psychiatrist, preferably using the patient's own words.

- What are your main problems or your main concerns?
- Specifically try to identify:
  - What is the nature of the problem?
  - Why and how has the individual presented this time?
  - What events led up to this presentation?

History of presenting complaints

- Identify specific symptoms that are present and their duration
  - *Chronological order:* What symptom started first?
  - *Onset and duration:* How did it start? Was it slowly, gradually, rapidly or suddenly? When did you last feel well?
  - *Course:* Did it get better, worse, remain the same, or was it up and down?
- Impairment in normal functioning (domestic, social and occupational functioning): the impact of symptoms on patient, family, work and social life
  - I would like to know how your problems have been affecting you, your family and your social life
  - How does it interfere with your normal life and activities?
- Recent stressors/stressful life events: note the time relationship between the onset of the current symptoms and the presence of social stressors/stressful life events
- Disturbance in biological symptoms
  - Sleep
  - Appetite
  - Libido
  - Weight
- Also obtain information about any treatments for their problem and the individual's response to treatment.

Screening questions: direct questioning

Start with open questions and then proceed to closed questions; and screen them for different types of symptom. (The questions to be asked under each category are discussed in detail in the Chapter 4.)

Box 1.1   Screening questions

- *Affective symptoms*—depression, mania
- *Suicidality*
- *Psychotic symptoms*—hallucinations, first-rank symptoms, delusions, negative symptoms
- *Neurotic symptoms*—anxiety, panic attacks, phobias, obsessions
- *Cognitive symptoms*—memory, confusion
- *Behavioural symptoms*—aggression, deliberate self-harm (DSH).

Past psychiatric history

- Have you ever had problems with your *mental health/nerves/depression*?
- Have you ever seen a psychiatrist before?
- Have you ever been admitted to a psychiatric hospital?
  - If so, ask about previous psychiatric episodes—the symptoms, complaints, precipitants, where they were seen, by whom, and the diagnosis, if known
- What *treatments* have you had before and what was the response?
  - Type of treatment-inpatient/outpatient, informal/detention
- Has there ever been a time when you felt completely well?
- Also ask about *inter-episode functioning* (psychiatric state between episodes—whether completely well or maintained on treatment)
- Have you ever attempted to harm yourself in the past? (history of overdoses, DSH or attempted suicide)

Past medical history

- Do you have any problems with your physical health?
- What about in the past? Any *medical* illnesses?
- Have you ever had any *operations* or been in the hospital?
- Have you ever had any *accidents, head injury or loss of consciousness*?

Current medications

- What medications do you take regularly?
- What medications have you had in the past?
- Are you allergic to any medications?

Family history

Now, I would like to ask you a few questions about yourself and your background.

Enquire about parents, siblings, grandparents, cousins, adoptive/foster/step-parents:

- Tell me about your parents? Your mum and dad . . .
  - How old are they?

- What did your parents work at?
- How did you get along with your parents?
- How did your parents get along together?
- Do you have any brothers or sisters; tell me about them?
- As far as you, know has anyone in your family or blood relatives ever had problems with their *mental health*?

Also, ask for history of suicides/alcoholism/epilepsy in the family.

Personal history

I would like to talk now about your childhood, education and adolescence.

Childhood

- Where were you born?
- Where were you brought up? And by whom?
- As far as you know was your mother's pregnancy normal?
- Was it a normal delivery?
- Were there any *problems* around the time of your birth or you growing up?
- Were you *walking and talking* at the correct times?
- Did you have any *serious illness as a young child*?
- When did you start school, and when did you finish school?
- Which schools did you go to?
- Did you enjoy school?
- Did you have any problems at school?
- Did you have many friends at school?
- Have you ever *been bullied* or *did you bully others*?
- Did you play *truant*? Were you ever *expelled* or *suspended* from school?
- When did you leave school?
- Did you gain any qualification at school?
- What did you do after finishing school? Did you go to college or university?
- Ask about college (subjects and qualifications) and other post-school training
- How would you *describe your childhood*?
- Ask in particular about:
  - Any *major loss* during childhood
  - *Separations*
  - Childhood *neglect*
  - *Physical/emotional/sexual abuses* in childhood
  - *Sibling rivalry.*

Work history

Enquire about the jobs held, nature of work, reasons for leaving jobs and any periods of unemployment?
- What did you work at? For how long? Then what happened?
- How many *steady jobs* did you have?
- What is your current job? How do you feel about your current job? Any problems with the job/colleagues?
- Are you unemployed at the moment? If so, why?

Psychosexual history

- Tell me about your partner/wife?
- How long have you been with your current partner?
- Are you married at present?
- How would you describe your marriage?
- How do you get on with her?
- Have you had any difficulties in your current relationship?
- Do you have children? If so, how many, and how old are they?
- How is your relationship with your children?
- How many previous relationships have you had?
- Tell me more about your previous relationships, previous partners/separations/divorces?

Current social circumstances

Social support

- Who lives at home with you at the moment?
- Do you have friends or family who live nearby?

Housing

- Type of accommodation:
  - Own/rented/council
  - Flat/house/bungalow
- How long have you been living there?

Finances and employment

- Employed/unemployed? Where do you work?

- What is your source of income?
- Enquire about income support/disability living allowance/state pension?
- Do you have any worries about debt or money in general?

Other support

Also enquire about other support such as community psychiatric nurse input, social workers' input, carer input, support workers, and voluntary agencies.

Drug and alcohol history

Enquire about smoking, alcohol and illicit drugs. If there is any positive history, explore further.

Smoking history

- Do you smoke?
- How much and how often in a day?
- Tell me more about it.

Alcohol history

- Do you drink alcohol?
- What do you usually drink?
- How often do you have a drink?
- How many drinks do you have on a typical day of drinking?
- What type of effect does alcohol have on you?
- How much money do you spend per day/week on drinking alcohol?
- When did it all start?
- How did you progress to the current level?
- Ask about details of treatment and details of any period of abstinence or binge drinking?
- Any detoxification programme? Was it completed?

Illicit drug history

- Have you ever used any recreational drugs such as cannabis, cocaine/crack, amphetamines, speed, ecstasy, LSD (or) acid? *Ask about individual drugs by naming them*
- What drugs are you using now?

- Tell me more about it
- How often do you take these drugs?
- What is the amount of drug taken?
- How much money do you spend in a day/week to get these drugs?
- What is the route of use—oral, smoked, snorted, injected? If drugs are injected, the following questions are useful:
  - Are needles used?
  - Where are they obtained?
  - Are needles shared?
  - What sites are used for injection?
- What effect is the patient seeking when using the drug?
- Ask whether more than one drug is used at a time
- How is the patient financing the drug use?

For more questions please see *Eliciting alcohol history and illicit drug history* in the Chapter 4.

Forensic history

- Have you ever been in trouble with the police or broken the law?
- Have you ever been charged or convicted of anything?
- Have you ever been involved with any criminal activity?
- If any, what are the offences/crimes that you have committed?
- Have you served any period in prison/probation/on remand?

Try to obtain a list of offences, charges, legal outcome and length and place of any prison sentence.

Premorbid personality

Start with open questions:

- How would you describe yourself as a person before you were ill?
- How do you think other people would describe you as a person?

Then ask closed questions about individual personality traits:

- Predominant mood
  - Optimistic/pessimistic
  - Stable/prone to anxiety
  - Cheerful/despondent

- Interpersonal relationships
  - Current friendships and relationships, previous relationships—ability to establish and maintain
  - Family relationships
- Coping strategies
  - When you find yourself in difficult situations, what do you do to cope?
  - What sort of things do you like to do to relax?
- Personal interests
  - Hobbies and interests
  - Use of leisure time
- Beliefs—religious beliefs
- Habits—food, fads etc.

Cluster A, Cluster B, Cluster C personality types—for more questions please see 'Eliciting premorbid personality' in Chapter 4.

Mental state examination

Appearance and behaviour

- Apparent age, stature, race
- Dressed, kempt, groomed
- Self-neglecting features
- Eye contact and rapport
- Posture, facial expression, mannerisms
- Prominent physical characteristics—scars, tattoos etc.
- Psychomotor changes, voluntary and involuntary movements, catatonic features.

Speech

- Rate
- Tone and volume
- Relevancy and coherency.

Mood

- Subjective mood—predominant mood in patient's own words
- Objective mood (your appraisal)—euthymic/euphoric/dysthymic/dysphoric, apprehensive/angry/apathetic.

Affect

- Labile, flat, blunt, reactive, congruent/incongruent.

Thought

- *Thought processes*
  - Logical, coherent and goal-directed
  - Loosening of association/blocking/perseveration
  - Tangentiality/circumstatiality/neologisms
- *Thought content*—mention only positive findings
  - Predominant topic or issue, preoccupations, ruminations
  - Unusual ideas or concerns
  - Obsessions, phobias and overvalued ideas
  - Ask specifically for *suicidal and/or homicidal ideation*—suicidal ideas/intentions/plans
  - Feelings of hopelessness or helplessness, ideas of worthlessness
- *Abnormal beliefs*
  - Delusions—content of any delusional system, its organization, the patient's convictions as to its validity and the type of delusions
  - Passivity phenomena.

Perception

- Illusions
- Hallucinations
- Depersonalization
- Derealization.

Cognition

Give a brief summary when all aspects of the cognitive state are normal; or a more detailed summary when some aspects are abnormal but not clinically decisive; or a full summary of testing when the results are diagnostically significant.

Orientation

- Time (day, date, year, time of the day)
- Place (name of the place/hospital/floor)
- Person.

Attention and concentration

- Subtracting a series of 7s from 100
- Days of the week forwards/backwards
- Months of the year forwards/backwards.

Memory

- Working memory—digit span 6 plus or minus 1
- Short-term memory—name and address: immediate and delayed (5-minute recall)
- Long-term memory
  - **Personal events:**
    a. When did you get married?
    b. When did you finish school?
  - **General events:**
    a. Who is the current prime minister of the UK?
    b. Who is the current president of the USA?
    c. What are the years of World War II?

Insight

- Recognition and attribution of illness
- Awareness of treatment that includes benefits of having the treatment and adherence/compliance to treatment.

Carry out a mini mental state examination, if required.

2

Physical examination

Aims of routine physical examination

- To assess the patient's baseline physical state
- To identify the presence or absence of any abnormal signs that could be associated with their physical or mental health condition
- To identify areas that require further examination, investigation and treatment.

Do not forget to mention this section even if there are no positive findings.

Try to look for relevant findings related to the psychiatric and medical history.

General examination

- Height and weight
- Bruises, scars, tattoos
- Any evidence of previous injury (e.g. self-cutting, etc.)
- Any signs of recent weight loss
- Any signs of physical neglect
- Vital signs:
  - Heart rate
  - Blood pressure
  - Respiratory rate
  - Temperature
  - Evidence of autonomic arousal, such as sweating, tremor or pallor.

Specific system examinations

These are to be done briefly. It is very important to examine what the history indicates is pertinent.

Remember to report the *positive findings*, if any, and important *negative findings* appropriate for your case.

The specific system examination should focus on the following:

- Cardiovascular examination
  - Blood pressure
  - Radial pulse-rate, rhythm and character
  - Heart sounds
  - Carotid bruits
  - Pedal edema
- Respiratory examination
  - Respiratory rate
  - Chest expansion
  - Percussion note
  - Auscultatory breath sounds
- Gastrointestinal examination
  - Any swelling, ascites or palpable masses
  - Bowel sounds
  - Hernias
- Central nervous system examination—*full neurological examination is the most important of all*
  - Examination of all four limbs for tone, power, reflexes, weakness and altered sensation
  - Gait inspection
  - Examination of hand-eye co-ordination
  - Check for involuntary movements
  - Cranial nerve examination
  - Fundoscopy
- Stigmata of *liver* disease—jaundice, spider naevi, gynaecomastia, palmar erythema, hepatomegaly
- Stigmata of *thyroid* disease
  - Hyperthyroidism—agitation, sweating, tremor, exophthalmos, lid-lag, pretibial myxoedema, thyroid bruit
  - Hypothyroidism—dry scaly skin, dry brittle hair, hair loss, goiter, hoarse voice, weight gain, sinus bradycardia, slow-relaxing reflexes, psycho-motor retardation

- Look for features of alcohol/drug intoxication and withdrawal features
  - *Features of alcohol withdrawal*—sweating, tremor, tachycardia, nausea, vomiting, generalized anxiety, psychomotor agitation, occasional visual, tactile or auditory hallucination
  - *Features of opiate withdrawal*—watering eyes and nose, yawning, nausea, vomiting, diarrhoea, tremor, joint pains, muscle cramps, sweating, dilated pupils, tachycardia, hypertension, and piloerection (goose-flesh)
- Extra-pyramidal side effects and other side effects of psychotropic medication
- Any other finding that is clearly relevant for your case—for example, in a patient with significant history of alcohol abuse, look for
  - Signs of alcohol withdrawal (tremor at rest, tachycardia, perspiration)
  - Signs of liver disease (jaundice, spider naevi, palmar erythema, hepatomegaly)
  - Neurological signs (ataxia, nystagmus, dysarthria and peripheral neuropathy).

Summary

Summary of positive findings and significant information relevant to the case obtained from history, mental state examination and physical examination.

3

Diagnosis and differential diagnoses

Diagnosis

All diagnostic features described below are based mainly on ICD-10 criteria.

Schizophrenia

A diagnosis of schizophrenia can be made if there is one clear symptom, or usually two or more symptoms if less clear cut, which should have been clearly present for most of the time during a period of *1 month or more.*

At least one of the following:

- Delusions of thought interference (thought withdrawal, thought insertion, thought broadcasting) or thought echo
- Delusions of control, influence or passivity; delusional perception
- Running commentary hallucinations; third-person hallucinations; hallucinations from part of the body
- Bizarre persistent delusions of other kinds that are culturally inappropriate and completely impossible.

A diagnosis of schizophrenia can also be made if symptoms from at least two of the groups listed below have been clearly present for most of the time during a period of *1 month or more.*

At least two of the following:

- Persistent hallucinations in any modality when accompanied by fleeting or half-formed delusions
- Breaks or interpolations in the train of thought leading to irrelevant, incoherent speech or neologisms
- Catatonic symptoms

- Negative symptoms
- A significant and consistent change in the overall quality of some aspects of the patient's behaviour.

If the symptoms are present for duration of less than one month it should be diagnosed in the first instance as acute schizophrenia-like psychotic disorder and should later be reclassified as schizophrenia if the symptoms persist for longer periods.

Paranoid schizophrenia

The general criteria for a diagnosis of schizophrenia must be satisfied. The clinical picture is often characterized by paranoid delusions (delusions of persecution, delusions of reference, control, passivity) usually accompanied by auditory hallucinations, other perceptual disturbances and hallucinations of the other modalities. In addition, disturbances of affect, volition, and speech may also be present.

Schizoaffective disorder

Schizoaffective disorder is characterized by having affective and schizophrenic symptoms, both prominent within the same episode of illness simultaneously or within a few days of each other, and they should be equally prominent.

It excludes patients with separate episodes of schizophrenia and affective disorders.

Mood-incongruent delusions or hallucinations in affective disorders do not justify a diagnosis of schizoaffective disorder.

Schizoaffective disorder, manic type

In this disorder, schizophrenic symptoms and manic symptoms are both prominent in the same episode of illness. There must be a prominent elevation of mood and at least one, and preferably two, schizophrenic symptoms as specified for schizophrenia should be clearly present.

Schizoaffective disorder, depressive type

In this disorder, schizophrenic symptoms and depressive symptoms are both prominent in the same episode of illness. There must be prominent depressive symptoms accompanied by at least two characteristic symptoms, and also at least one, or preferably two, schizophrenic symptoms as specified for schizophrenia should be clearly present.

Schizoaffective disorder, mixed type

Here, symptoms of schizophrenia coexist with those of a mixed bipolar affective disorder.

Persistent delusional disorder

- Circumscribed symptoms of non-bizarre delusions
- Absence of prominent hallucinations
- No evidence of thought disorder or mood disorder
- Symptoms should have been present for at least 3 months.

Depression

Typical symptoms:

- Depressed mood
- Anhedonia (loss of interest and enjoyment)
- Reduced energy leading to increased fatigueability and diminished activity.

Core symptoms:

- Poor memory, reduced attention and concentration
- Low self-esteem, reduced self confidence
- Ideas of guilt, bleak and pessimistic views of the future, unworthiness
- Ideas or acts of self-harm or suicide
- Disturbed sleep
- Diminished appetite.

Classification:

- Mild depressive episode—at least two of the typical symptoms plus at least two of the core symptoms
- Moderate depressive episode—at least two of the typical symptoms should be present plus at least three, and preferably four, of the core symptoms
- Severe depressive episode—all three of the typical symptoms should be present plus at least four of the core symptoms, some of which should be of severe intensity.

Step 1: Decide if mild, moderate or severe and also assess the degree of functional impairment

For depressive episodes, a duration of *at least 2 weeks* is usually required for diagnosis, but if the symptoms are particularly severe and of very rapid onset, it may be justified to make this diagnosis after less than 2 weeks.

The differentiation between the three grades rests upon a complicated clinical judgement that involves the *number, type and severity* of symptoms present plus the extent of impairment in social and work activities.

Step 2: Somatic syndrome present/absent

Somatic symptoms:

- Loss of interest or pleasure in activities that are usually enjoyable
- Early morning awakening; at least 2 hours before the usual time
- Diurnal variation of mood, being worst in the morning
- Weight loss (5% or more of body weight in the last month)
- Marked loss of appetite
- Marked loss of libido
- Objective evidence of definite psychomotor retardation or agitation.

With somatic syndrome, four or more of the somatic symptoms should be present.

The use of this category may be justified if only two or three somatic symptoms are present, but they are unusually severe.

It is presumed that the somatic syndrome will almost always be present in a severe depressive episode.

Step 3: Psychotic symptoms present/absent

Psychotic symptoms involve a severe depressive episode in which delusions, hallucinations or depressive stupor are present and the delusions or hallucinations may be specified as mood congruent or mood incongruent.

Step 4: Assess suicidality

Assess suicidality of a patient presenting with low mood.

Recurrent depressive disorder

The disorder is characterized by repeated episodes of depression without any history of independent episodes of mood elevation and overactivity that fulfill the criteria of mania.

It occurs in the following forms:

- Recurrent depressive disorder, current episode mild, with/without somatic syndrome

- Recurrent depressive disorder, current episode moderate, with/without somatic syndrome
- Recurrent depressive disorder, current episode severe without psychotic symptoms
- Recurrent depressive disorder, current episode severe with psychotic symptoms.

Mania

Decide if hypomania or mania with/ without psychotic symptoms.

Hypomania

- Persistent mild elation of mood (for at least several days on end)
- Increased energy and activity
- Marked feelings of well-being, both physical and mental efficiency
- Over familiarity, talkativeness, increased sociability
- Increased sexual energy and decreased need for sleep
- Impaired attention and concentration
- Mild overspending and development of new interests.

In hypomania, the symptoms are often present but not to the extent that they lead to severe disruption of work or social functioning.

Mania (without psychotic symptoms)

- Elevated mood, (not in keeping with the individual's circumstance)
- Increased energy resulting in overactivity
- Disinhibition, excessive spending
- Accelerated thoughts and pressure of speech
- Decreased need for sleep, appetite disturbance, increased libido
- Distractibility, impaired attention and concentration
- Inflated self-esteem and grandiose or freely expressed overoptimistic ideas.

The episode should last for 1 week and should be severe enough to disrupt social or occupational life more or less completely.

Mania (with psychotic symptoms)

- The clinical picture is that of a more severe form of mania
- Delusions—delusions of persecution, delusions of grandiosity, religious delusions

- Delusions or hallucinations can be specified as mood congruent or mood incongruent.

Bipolar affective disorder

Bipolar affective disorder is characterized by repeated episodes (at least two) of hypomania/mania and depression, and the recovery is complete between the episodes.

Bipolar affective disorder, hypomania

The present episode should fulfill the criteria for hypomania, and there must have been at least one other affective episode in the past (hypomania, mania, depression or mixed).

Bipolar affective disorder, manic without psychotic symptoms

The present episode should fulfill the criteria for mania without psychotic symptoms, and there must have been at least one other affective episode in the past (hypomania, mania, depression or mixed).

Bipolar affective disorder, manic with psychotic symptoms

The present episode should fulfill the criteria for mania with psychotic symptoms, and there must have been at least one other affective episode in the past (hypomania, mania, depression or mixed).

Bipolar affective disorder, current episode mild or moderate depression

The present episode should fulfill the criteria for a depressive episode of either mild or moderate severity, and there must have been at least one other affective episode in the past (hypomania, mania, depression or mixed).

Bipolar affective disorder, current episode severe depression without psychotic symptoms

The present episode should fulfill the criteria for a severe depressive episode without psychotic symptoms, and there must have been at least one other affective episode in the past (hypomania, mania, depression or mixed).

Bipolar affective disorder, current episode severe depression with psychotic symptoms

The present episode should fulfill the criteria for a severe depressive episode with psychotic symptoms, and there must have been at least one other affective episode in the past (hypomania, mania, depression or mixed).

Bipolar affective disorder, current episode mixed

The patient has had at least one hypomania, manic or mixed affective episode in the past and currently exhibits both manic and depressive symptoms, both prominent for the greater part of the current episode, and that the episode has lasted for at least 2 weeks.

Generalized anxiety disorder

At least four of the following types of symptom should be present, and the symptoms should be present most days for at least 6 months:

- Autonomic arousal: palpitations, tachycardia, sweating, dry mouth, trembling and shaking
- Physical symptoms: difficulty in breathing, chest pain/discomfort, choking sensation, nausea and abdominal distress, difficulty swallowing
- Mental state symptoms: dizziness, light-headedness, fear of losing control, fear of dying or fear of 'going crazy'
- General symptoms: numbness, tingling sensations and hot flushes
- Symptoms of tension: muscular tension, aches and pains, feeling 'on the edge', inability to relax
- Others: exaggerated startle response, persistent irritability, concentration difficulties and difficulty getting to sleep.

Agoraphobia with (or without) panic disorder

Diagnosis in ICD-10:

- Symptoms of anxiety (all including psychological, behavioural and autonomic symptoms) should be present, and they are not secondary to other symptoms, delusions or obsessions
- Anxiety occurs in at least two of the following situations: crowds, public places, travelling alone and travelling away from home
- Avoidance behaviour: avoidance of the phobic situation as a prominent feature.

Social phobia

- Symptoms of anxiety (all including psychological, behavioural and autonomic symptoms) should be present, and they are not secondary to other symptoms delusions or obsessions
- Anxiety occurs particularly in social situations (restricted to eating in public, public speaking, encounters with the opposite sex)
- Avoidance behaviour: avoidance of the phobic situation as a prominent feature. There may be associated blushing, nausea and hand tremor, often leading to avoidance behaviour and alcohol misuse.

Specific phobia

- Symptoms of anxiety (all including psychological, behavioural and autonomic symptoms) should be present, and they are not secondary to other symptoms delusions or obsessions
- The anxiety must be restricted to the presence of the particular phobic object or situation.
- Avoidance behaviour: avoidance of the phobic situation as a prominent feature. There may be associated blushing, nausea and hand tremor, often leading to avoidance behaviour and alcohol misuse.

Panic disorder (episodic paroxysmal anxiety)

Essential features are recurrent; unpredictable attacks of panic in a range of situations.

Diagnosis in ICD -10:

- Several severe attacks within the last month:
  - In circumstances where there is no objective danger
  - Not confined to known or predictable situations
- Freedom from anxiety symptoms between attacks.

Obsessive-compulsive disorder

Symptoms (obsessional symptoms or compulsive acts) must be present on most days over the preceding 2 weeks, causing distress and interference with normal activities.

- Recognized as the individual's own thoughts or impulses
- Resistance: there must be at least one thought or act that is still resisted unsuccessfully

- Ritual is not in itself pleasurable
- Thoughts, images or impulses must be unpleasantly repetitive.

Post-traumatic stress disorder

- Extreme nature of traumatic event
- The onset follows the trauma with a latency period which may range from a few weeks to months but rarely exceeds 6 months.
- Symptoms of increased psychological sensitivity and arousal: difficulty in concentration, irritability, sleep disturbances, exaggerated startle response and hypervigilance
- Persistent reliving of the event in recurring dreams, nightmares, vivid memories and flashbacks
- Avoidance: actual or preferred avoidance of situations/circumstances associated with the stressor, which are a reminder of the event
- Disinterest, detachment and numbness.

Adjustment disorder

- Onset within 1 month of stressful event or life change
- The duration of symptoms does not usually exceed 6 months.
- States of subjective distress and emotional disturbance, usually interfering with normal social functioning and performance, and arising in the period of adaptation to a significant life changer to the consequences of a stressful life event (including the presence or possibility of serious physical illness).

Anorexia nervosa

- Weight loss >15% of total body weight and below-expected body mass index (BMI) of 17.5 or less
- Body image distortion—fear of fatness held as an overvalued idea
- Avoidance of fattening foods, with behaviours aimed at losing weight, such as vomiting, purging, over exercise and use of appetite suppressants
- Amenorrhoea, reduced sexual interest, impotence
- Pubertal delay if onset is early.

Bulimia nervosa

- Persistent preoccupation with food and irresistible craving for food
- Binges—episodes of overeating

- Avoidance of fattening foods, with behaviours aimed at losing weight such as vomiting, purging, over exercise and use of appetite suppressants
- Morbid fear of fatness with imposed 'low weight threshold'.

Alcohol/drug dependence syndrome

Edwards and Gross criteria 1976:

- Loss of control of consumption
- Increased tolerance to the effects of drugs
- Signs of withdrawal on attempted abstinence
- Relief of withdrawal symptoms by drinking or by taking drugs
- Rapid reinstatement of previous pattern of drug use after abstinence
- Continued use despite negative consequences
- Narrowing of the drinking/drug-taking repertoire
- Primacy of drug-seeking behaviour.

Dementia in Alzheimer's disease

- Global deterioration in intellectual capacity and disturbance in higher cortical functions, such as memory, thinking, orientation, comprehension, calculation, language, learning abilities and judgement; an appreciable decline in intellectual functioning and some interference with personal activities of daily living
- Insidious onset with slow deterioration
- Absence of clinical evidence or findings from special investigations suggestive of organic brain disease or other systemic abnormalities
- Absence of sudden onset or physical/neurological signs.

Vascular dementia

- Impairment of congnitive function such as memory loss and intellectual impairment
- Onset may be gradual as in some subtypes, or, can be abrupt following one particular ischaemic episode
- Stepwise deterioratism
- Presence of focal neurological signs and symptoms
- Relative preservation of personality and insight

Lewy Body Dementia

- Fluctuating cognitive impairment affecting both memory and higher cortical functions; the fluctuation is pronounced with both episodic confusion and lucid intervals as in delirium

- Prominent visual hallucinations and/or auditory hallucinations usually accompanied by secondary paranoid delusions and the whole spectrum of psychiatric presentations can also occur
- Motor features of parkinsonism
- Neuroleptic sensitivity – exaggerated form of response to standard doses of neuroleptics
- Repeated unexplained falls

Note: If both motor and cognitive symptoms develop within 12 months, it is conventional to give a diagnosis of Lewy body dementia. A diagnosis of Parkinson's disease dementia is given if the parkinsonian symptoms have existed for at least 12 months before dementia develops and the dementing process develops in the course of established Parkinson's disease.

Emotionally unstable personality disorder

Borderline type

- Boredom and chronic emptiness
- Identity confusion
- Recurrent suicide threats or acts of self-harm
- Impulsivity
- Relationship difficulties—intense and unstable relationships
- Affective instability—unpredictable affect.

Impulsive type

- Inability to control anger
- Unpredictable affect and behaviour.

Differential diagnosis

Work out the differential diagnosis by applying the *diagnostic hierarchy* and process of exclusion.

- Organic illness, epilepsy, drug- and alcohol-induced illness
- Schizophrenia and other psychotic disorders
- Affective disorders
- Neurotic disorders, eating disorders, post-traumatic stress disorder (PTSD), somatization disorders
- Personality traits/disorders.

Useful hints

- Know the ICD-10 well as it is the basis for differential diagnosis. You should, therefore, familiarize yourself with this classification, and it can be very helpful to have pre-prepared a list of standardized differential diagnoses for the common presenting problems that we come across in our day-to-day practice
- Many examiners may not be familiar with DSM-4 and the advantages of DSM-4 for measurement seldom apply
- It is useful to make an introductory statement that '*According to ICD-10, my differential diagnosis is ...*'. For example, recurrent depressive disorder, current episode moderate with somatic syndrome
- Proceed as follows:
  - Prepare a *list* of all the diagnoses you wish to present
  - Give the reasons *for* and *against* each diagnosis
  - Make clear which are *competing* diagnoses (i.e., the main differentials) and which are *additional* diagnoses, e.g., severe depression with psychotic symptoms, with a number of competing diagnostic possibilities as well as alcohol dependence and a dependent personality
  - Also make clear if you consider one (or more than one) diagnosis is clearly preferable
  - Carefully review organic possibilities (such as withdrawal from substance misuse) and include them wherever there is some clinical indication
  - Only state actual possibilities, and if you are really considering them in the differential for your particular case, be prepared to justify your reasons.

Here below, I have discussed in detail, the differential diagnoses of common psychiatric conditions seen in clinical practice and in exam conditions.

Schizoprenia

- Organic psychotic disorder:
  - Drug-induced psychosis; related to substance misuse, drug intoxication and withdrawal with stimulants (cannabis, cocaine, LSD, amphetamine and ecstasy)
  - Delirium
  - Related to a general medical condition
- Schizoaffective disorder
- Bipolar affective disorder manic episode with psychotic symptoms
- Depressive episode with psychotic symptoms
- Delusional disorder
- Acute and transient psychotic disorder
- Paranoid personality disorder.

Medical conditions to be excluded when evaluating a patient with first episode psychosis include:

- Temporal lobe epilepsy
- Toxic drug reaction
- Systemic lupus erythematosus
- Infections—limbic encephalitis, subacute sclerosing encephalitis, neurosyphilis and HIV disease
- CNS neoplasm, cerebral trauma
- Cerebrovascular disease (late-onset schizophrenia)
- Huntington's disease
- Metabolic disorders—electrolyte imbalance, hypoglycaemia, hepatic or renal disease
- Endocrine disorders—hyper- and hypothyroidism, Addison's disease, hyper- and hypoparathyroidism
- Demyelinating disease, such as multiple sclerosis and metachromatic dystrophy.

Persistent delusional disorder

- Rule out physical causes, e.g., head injury, epilepsy, CNS infection
- Substance-induced delusional disorder, e.g., alcohol, hallucinogens, stimulants
- Schizophrenia
- Mood disorder with delusions
- Elderly patients (late paraphrenia)
- Paranoid personality disorder
- Obsessive-compulsive disorder
- Body dysmorphic disorder
- Hypochondriasis.

Mania

- Schizophrenia
- Schizoaffective disorder
- Drug or alcohol induced mania
- Medical disorder induced mania
- Delirium or acute confusional state
- Agitated depression in the elderly
- Obsessive-compulsive disorder (OCD) or other anxiety disorders

- Circadian rhythm disorders
- Puerperal psychosis (in women)
- Dementia, especially frontal (in the elderly).

Organic causes of manic and hypomanic symptoms:

- Metabolic disturbance—postoperative states, postinfection states, hyperthyroidism, Cushing's disease, Addison's disease
- Infection—influenza, neurosyphilis, AIDS (HIV), herpes simplex encephalitis
- Neurological conditions—epilepsy, post-cerebrovascular accident, multiple sclerosis, right temporal seizure focus
- Neoplasm—parasagittal meningioma, suprasellar craniopharyngioma, tumour of the floor of the fourth ventricle
- Drugs associated with manic symptoms—amphetamines, cocaine, hallucinogens and opiates
- Medications associated with manic symptoms—antidepressants, isoniazid, levodopa, methyl phenidate hydrochloride, procyclidine hydrochloride, bromocriptine mesilate, corticosteroids, cimetidine, ciclosporin

Depression

- Mood disorder due to a general medical condition
- Substance-induced mood disorder—alcohol, amphetamine, heroin, cocaine, etc.
- Bipolar affective disorder
- Dysthymia
- Consider stress-related disorders, such as adjustment disorder, grief reaction, PTSD
- Dementia
- Anxiety disorders, such as social phobias, OCD, panic disorder
- Schizophrenia (negative symptoms)
- Personality disorders, such as borderline PD.

Medical conditions inducing mood disorder:

- Metabolic: iron-deficiency anaemia, niacin deficiency (pellagra), hypercalcaemia
- Infective: encephalitis, post-viral, hepatitis, infectious mononucleosis, HIV
- Neurological: post-stroke, Parkinson's disease, multiple sclerosis, intracranial tumours (e.g., frontal)
- Non-metastasis manifestation of neoplasm, e.g., pancreatic carcinoma

- Endocrine disorders: hypothyroidism, Cushing's syndrome, Addison's disease hyperparathyroidism
- Iatrogenic: reserpine, propranolol hydrochloride, alpha methyldopa, corticosteroids, effects of chemotherapeutic agents, such as vincristine sulphate and interferons, whole-brain radiotherapy.

Anxiety disorders

- Medical disorders causing anxiety symptoms—thyrotoxicosis, hypoglycaemia, pheochromocytoma, temporal lobe epilepsy, anaemia, asthma, cardiac arrhythmias and carcinoid tumours, hypoxia and sepsis
- Medication inducing anxiety symptoms—bronchodilators, antihypertensives, antiarrhythmics, anticonvulsants, levothyroxine, antiparkinsonian agents, antidepressants, antipsychotics, Antabuse (disulfiram) reactions
- Affective disorder—depression, depression with agitated features
- Consider all other anxiety disorders—agoraphobia, social phobia, specific phobia, panic disorder, generalized anxiety disorder, mixed anxiety and depressive disorder, obsessive-compulsive disorder, acute stress reaction, PTSD, adjustment reaction
- Substance misuse—alcohol withdrawal symptoms, drug withdrawal symptoms
- Prodromal symptom of schizophrenia
- Early stage of dementia.

Social phobias

- Agoraphobias
- Panic disorder
- Depressive disorder
- Generalized anxiety disorder
- Avoidant personality disorder
- Social inadequacy
- Schizophrenia.

Obsessive-compulsive disorder

- Normal thoughts, worries (but recurrent)
- Anankastic personality disorder
- Depressive disorder
- Hypochondriasis
- Phobias

- Schizophrenia
- Body dysmorphic disorder

Post-traumatic stress disorder

- Adjustment disorder
- Acute stress reaction
- Enduring personality change after a catastrophic event
- Depressive/mood disorder
- Generalized anxiety disorders
- Phobias
- Panic disorder
- Substance-induced disorders
- Obsessive-compulsive disorder
- Schizophrenia or other associated psychosis.

Anorexia nervosa

- Weight loss due to a general medical condition: especially gastrointestinal (GI) disorders, such as inflammatory bowel disease, malabsorption syndrome and occult malignancy
- Vomiting secondary to gastric outlet obstruction
- Brain tumour
- HIV
- Loss of appetite may be secondary to drugs, e.g., selective serotonin (5-hydroxytryptamine) reuptake inhibitors (SSRIs), amphetamines
- Bulimia nervosa (50% of anorexia suffers also meet the criteria for bulimia nervosa)
- Depressive disorder
- Obsessive-compulsive disorder
- Schizophrenia.

Bulimia nervosa

- Upper GI disorders
- Depressive disorder
- Obsessive-compulsive disorder
- Personality disorders
- Drug-related increased appetite (antipsychotics, antidepressants especially tricyclic antidepressants, mood stabilizers)
- Causes of recurrent overeating, such as Kleine-Levin syndrome.

Dementia

- Depressive disorder (pseudo-dementia)
- Delirium
- Drugs
- Amnesic syndromes
- Learning disability
- Late-onset psychotic disorder
- Normal ageing.

Alzheimer's dementia

- Non-Alzheimer's dementia
- Vascular dementia/multi-infarct dementia
- Lewy body dementia
- Fronto-temporal dementia
- Subcortical dementias, such as Parkinson's disease, Huntington's disease
- Metabolic toxic dementias, such as hypothyroidism, hyperparathyroidism, vitamin B12 and folate deficiency
- Infections, such as syphilis, HIV or chronic meningitis.

Schizotypal disorder

- Autism
- Asperger's syndrome
- Chronic substance misuse
- Personality disorders, such as schizoid, paranoid and borderline types
- Expressive language disorder.

Asperger's syndrome

- Schizophrenia—paranoid, simple
- Personality disorders—schizoid, avoidant, anankastic and dissocial
- Attention deficit hyperactivity disorders
- Anxiety states—selective mutism, social phobias, panic disorder, generalized anxiety disorders
- Obsessive-compulsive disorder.

Borderline personality disorder

- Organic personality disorder—secondary to a general medical condition, e.g., cerebral neoplasms especially in frontal and parietal lobes

- Mood disorders—depressive disorder with atypical features
- Psychotic disorders
- Other personality disorders, such as antisocial PD, histrionic PD, dependent PD types.

4

Observed interview tasks

You will be asked to interview the patient on one or two areas from the history or the mental state, occupying 10 minutes, which must be planned and practiced carefully.

The aim is to carry out the tasks set and to demonstrate essential clinical interviewing skills. These can be roughly divided into those of empathy and control.

Suggested approach

- Greet and introduce the patient to the examiners
- The purpose of the interview should be explained briefly—it is essential to give a clear framework of what the interview will be about, in words that the patient will understand
- Obtain permission before you proceed
- It is essential at the beginning of the task to give priority to the patient's feelings and attitudes and not to the strict definition of the task
- Start with **open** questions and then proceed to **closed** questions
- Establishing control needs to follow empathy
- At the end of the interview thank the patient.

The following sections give some of the frequently asked tasks in the exam.

Eliciting alcohol history

TASK: Explore the following—current usage, longitudinal history and features of dependence syndrome (Edwards and Gross criteria)

Edwards and Gross' alcohol dependence syndrome (1976)

- Subjective awareness of the compulsion to drink
- Increased tolerance
- Withdrawal symptoms
- Salience of drinking behaviour
- Reinstatement after abstinence
- Narrowing of drinking repertoire
- Relief drinking.

Questions

- Current usage in a typical day/week
  - Do you drink alcohol at all?
  - What do you usually drink?
  - How often do you have a drink?
  - Describe a typical day for me. Could you describe any pattern?
  - How many drinks do you have on a typical day of drinking?
  - What sort of effect does alcohol have on you?
- Longitudinal history
  - When did it all start?
  - What was the first drink?
  - With whom did you have the first drink?
  - Was it of your own free will (or) peer pressure?
  - How did you progress to the current level?
    a. Started drinking occasionally (social drink)
    b. Regular weekend drinking
  - How much would you drink at the weekend?
  - Do you drink during the week?
    a. Regular evening drinking
    b. Regular lunchtime drinking
    c. Early morning drinking (progressive)
  - What did you used to drink in the past? And what do you drink now?

Edwards and Gross criteria for dependence syndrome

- Compulsion
  - Do you sometimes crave a drink?
  - Do you have a compulsive urge to drink?
- Tolerance
  - Does a drink have less of an effect on you than before?
  - Nowadays, do you need more alcohol to get drunk than you needed before?
- Withdrawal symptoms
  - What happens if you go without a drink for a day or two?
  - Have you ever had 'the shakes'?
  - If you don't drink for a day or two, do you experience any withdrawal symptoms such as sweating, shaking, weakness, headaches, feeling sick or pounding in your heart?
- Relief drinking
  - Do you need a drink first thing in the morning to steady your nerves?
  - Do you have to gulp the first few drinks of the day?
- Stereotyped pattern
  - Do you always drink in the same pub?
  - Do you always drink with the same company?
- Treatment and rapid reinstatement
  - Ask about details of treatment and details of any period of abstinence or binge drinking
  - What helped you keep off drink?
  - Have you ever had an extended period of time when you didn't drink?
  - What happened to make you start drinking again?
  - Have you ever gone to anyone for help with your drink problem?
  - Have you ever been in hospital because of your drinking?
  - Any detoxification programme?
    a. Was it completed or not?
    b. If not, what are the reasons?
- Primacy
  - How important is drink compared with other activities?
  - How often do you miss family and social commitments because of drinking?
  - Have you been giving primary importance to alcohol, and have you been neglecting other alternative pleasures or interests?

TASK: Elicit the complications following alcohol misuse and assess insight and motivation

Physical health problems

- What do you think are the consequences of your drinking?
- Have you ever had any health problems due to drinking?
- Ask specific questions about:
  - Accidents and head injury
  - Memory problems
  - Blackouts, falls, fits.

Mental health problems

- Have you ever had severe shaking, heard voices and seen things that were not there after heavy drinking?
- Also ask specifically about:
  - Anxiety, depression
  - Suicidal ideation/behaviour.

Social problems

- Relationship difficulties with the partner, children, family members and friends.
  - Has your drinking ever led to problems with your family, friends, work or the police?
  - How has it affected your family life—rows or arguments with friends or family?
- Problems at the work place
  - Has your drinking had an effect on your job, e.g., missing work, late arrival, Monday absences?
- Financial problems
  - Have you ever had any financial problems because of your habit?

Legal problems

- Drink driving, drunk and disorderly behaviour, fights while drunk
  - Have you actually had an accident or hurt yourself?
  - Have you ever been arrested because of your drinking?
  - Have you ever been convicted of drink driving?

Insight and motivation

- Do you think that the problems you experience currently are related in any way to your drinking?
- What makes you feel that way and could you please explain that?
- Do you feel that you have a problem with alcohol?
- What would you like to do?
- Have you ever thought of giving it up completely?
- What do you think will happen if you give up completely?

Eliciting illicit drug history

TASK: Elicit illicit drug history looking for features of drug dependence and complications experienced

Open questions

- Are there any tablets or medicines that you take apart from those you get from your doctor?
- Is there anything that you buy from the chemists or get from friends?
- Have you ever used any recreational drugs or illegal drugs such as cannabis, cocaine/crack, amphetamines, speed, ecstasy, LSD or acid? (Ask about individual drugs by naming them)
- What about tablets to 'settle your nerves' or to help you sleep?

Current usage

- What drugs are you using now?
- What is the frequency of use?
- What is the pattern of typical drug using?
- What is the amount of drug taken? (in appropriate measures)
- What effect are you seeking when using the drug?
- How much money do you spend in a day/week to get these drugs?
- What is the route of use—oral, smoked, snorted, injected? If injected, the following questions are useful to ask:
  - Are needles used?
  - Where are they obtained?
  - Are needles shared?
  - What sites are used for injection?
- What risky behaviour does the patient engage in?
  - Injecting and sharing needles?

- Unsafe sex?
- Sex for drugs?
- Is more than one drug used at a time?
- How is he/she financing the drug use?

Longitudinal history

Ask about the patient's age at first use of drugs, and when the patient started to use the drug regularly.

- When did it start?
- What was the first drug taken?
- Was it by your own free will or peer pressure?
- How did you progress to the current level?

Features of 'dependence syndrome'

- Compulsion
  - Do you sometimes crave for drugs?
  - Do you have a compulsive urge to take drugs?
- Tolerance
  - Do you have to increase the amount of drugs that you take to get the same effect?
  - Does the same amount give you less of an effect than it used to?
- Withdrawal symptoms
  - If you don't take drugs for a day or two, do you experience any withdrawal symptoms? For example, if the patient takes heroin, ask about symptoms such as sweating, gooseflesh, running nose, watery eyes, etc.
  - Ask the patient to describe any withdrawal symptoms in their own words
- Complications
  - Have you experienced any complications? (Ask about physical, mental and social complications?
  - Have you ever worried about:
    a. Hepatitis B or C and HIV?
    b. Complications of injecting like infections, abscesses, septicaemia?
    c. Accidents, head injury, falls, fits?
    d. Anxiety, depression, hearing voices, seeing things?
    e. Financial problems?
    f. Arguments with friends or family members or work colleagues?
- Treatment
  - What is patient's past experience of treatment for a drug problem?
  - Have you ever gone to anyone for help to come out of this?

- Have you ever been in hospital for a drug problem?
- Have there been any periods of abstinence when you were not using any drugs and if so, what has helped you achieve this?
- What triggers have brought on this habit again?

Eliciting post-traumatic stress disorder history

TASK: Explore the following—details of the traumatic incident/accident itself and core features of post-traumatic stress disorder

Traumatic incident

Explore the details of the accident, in particular the perceived severity and establish the level of distress and fear at the time of the event. Here, approach the patient *empathetically* as it is difficult to talk about traumatic incidents, and acknowledge the patient's distress.

- Could you describe the accident please?
- Find out about when it happened, how terrifying it was?
- Ask about any injuries, in particular, head injury, loss of consciousness, whether any other person was injured etc.
- Enquire about any blame, litigation, court cases and their outcome.

Core features

Core features of post-traumatic stress disorder are intrusions, avoidance, hyperarousal and emotional detachment and numbness.

- Intrusions
  - How often do you think about the accident?
  - Do you sometimes feel as if the accident is happening again?
  - Do you get flashbacks?
  - Have you revisited the scene?
  - Do you get any distressing dreams/nightmares of the event?
  - What happens if you hear about an accident?
- Avoidance
  - How hard is it for you to talk about the accident?
  - Have you been to the place where the accident happened?
  - Do you deliberately try to avoid thinking about accidents?
  - Do you make any effort to avoid the thoughts or conversations associated with the trauma? How would you do that?

- Do you make any effort to avoid activities, places or people that arouse recollection of the trauma?
- Hyperarousal
  - Have you had the feeling that you are always on the edge?
  - Do you tend to worry a lot about things going wrong? (feeling anxious)
  - Do you startle easily? (Enhanced startle response)
  - Tell me about your sleep please (explore for sleep disturbance)
  - Are you sometimes afraid to go to sleep?
  - How has your concentration been recently?
  - How has your memory been lately?
  - Tell me about your temper please (irritability)
- Emotional detachment and numbness
  - How do you feel in yourself generally?
  - Have there been any changes in your feelings generally? (emotional detachment)
  - How do you see the future?

Other issues

- Assess the mode of onset of symptoms, duration, progress, severity and frequency of current symptoms
- Distress and impairment of social functioning
  - I would like to know how your problems have been affecting you, your family and your social life
- Explore co-morbidity
  - Mood symptoms, especially depression and anxiety symptoms
  - Current coping mechanisms, including drugs and alcohol.

Eliciting eating disorder history

TASK: Elicit history with a view to exploring the psychological issues and abnormal eating pattern

Psychological issues

- Do you think you have a problem with your weight and eating?
- How do you feel about your weight right now?
- What is your ideal weight?
- Why is this weight ideal for you?
- Are you satisfied with how you look?
- Do you feel fat? Do you feel ugly?

- How do you feel when you see your image in a mirror?
- Do you feel that you have a distorted body image? If so, in what way?
- Do you fear loss of control? What do you mean by that?
- What do you feel would happen if you did not control your weight or eating?

Eating issues

- What is a typical day's eating?
- Is there a pattern? Does it vary?
- Do you avoid any particular foods? And if so, why?
- Do you restrict fluids?
- *Binge eating*
    - Do you ever have times where you feel that your eating is out of control or seems excessive?
    - Do you ever binge eat? (i.e., eat, during a short space of time, quantities of food that are definitely larger than most people would eat during a similar time and in similar circumstances)
    - When did you first start binge eating?
    - How often do you do it and why do you binge eat?
    - Tell me about a typical binge? (obtain information about type of foods eaten, quantity of food, duration of the binge, vomiting or purging after the binge)
    - How do you feel just before you binge?
    - Can you identify any particular cause (e.g., feelings, stressors, social situations) that may trigger the binge?
    - How do you feel while you are binge eating?
    - How do you feel after bingeing?
- *Vomiting*
    - Have you ever had to make yourself sick? If so how?
    - How often do you do this?
    - Can you tell me why you make yourself vomit?
- *Laxatives, diuretics, emetics, appetite suppressants, exercise*
    - Often, many people with these problems use other methods to control their weight such as (give examples and ask specifically) taking laxatives, water pills, emetics and appetite suppressants?
    - For what reason do you use it?
    - Do you fast for a day or more?
    - Do you exercise?
    - How often do you exercise?
    - Is this to burn off calories?
    - Do you use exercise as a means of controlling your weight?

Physical symptoms

- Menstrual changes
  - When was your last period?
  - Are you menstruating regularly?
- Changes in libido
- Symptoms of anaemia: weakness, lethargy, constipation
  - Do you feel the cold badly?
  - Have you noticed any weakness in your muscles?
  - Have you fainted or had dizzy spells?
  - Have you noticed any palpitations?

Other issues

Explore:

- Any difficult situation at home or at work
- Current relationship
- Social activities and life in general
- Recent stressors.

Eliciting symptoms of depression

TASK: Elicit the features of depression

Eliciting symptoms of depression and suicidality

- How are you feeling in yourself?
- How bad has it been?
- Have you cried at all?
- If I were to ask you to rate your mood, on a scale of 0 to 10 where 0 is the rock bottom of how you feel, and 10 is the best of your spirits, where would you place your mood over the last couple of weeks?
- Can you enjoy anything?
- What are the things that you find enjoyable/interesting?
- Is the level of enjoyment same as before?
- Have you lost enjoyment for things you used to enjoy?
- How have you been in your energy levels these days?
- Have you been feeling drained of energy lately?
- Have you wanted to stay away from other people?
- How do you spend your day?

Eliciting biological symptoms

- How has your sleep been recently?
- Do you need less sleep than usual?
- Have you had any trouble getting off to sleep?
- Do you wake early in the morning?
- Is your depression/mood worse at any particular time of day?
- What is the best time/worst time of the day for you?
- What has your appetite been like recently?
- Have you lost any weight lately?
- Has there been any change in your interest in sex?

Cognitive symptoms

- How has your concentration been lately?
- How has been your memory recently?
- How confident do you feel in yourself?
- How do you describe your self-esteem to be?

Eliciting suicidal intent and negative thoughts

- Have you felt that life wasn't worth living?
- How do you see the future?
- Do you feel inferior to others or even worthless?
- Do you feel hopeless about yourself? Has life seemed quite hopeless?
- Do you feel helpless?
- Do you feel that life is a burden?
- Do you wish yourself dead? Why do you feel this way?
- Have you ever felt like 'ending it all'?
- Did you actually try?
- How do you feel about it now?
- Would you do anything to harm yourself or to hurt yourself?
- Have you got any plans to end your life? What plans?

Eliciting feelings of guilt

- Do you feel that you've done something wrong?
- Do you feel guilty about things?
- Do you tend to blame yourself at all?
- Do you tend to blame anyone else for your problems?
- Do you have any regrets?

- Do you feel that you've committed a crime, or sinned greatly or deserve punishment?

Duration, course, effects, coping

- How long have you been feeling like this?
- What do you think might have caused this?
- How is it affecting your life?
- How do you manage to cope?
- Do you get any help?

Eliciting manic/hypomanic symptoms

TASK: Elicit the features of mania/hypomania

Core features of manic/hypomanic symptoms

- How are you feeling in yourself?
- Have you sometimes felt unusually/particularly cheerful and 'on top of the world', without any reason?
- How is your energy level?
- Do you find yourself extremely active but not getting tired?
- Have you felt particularly full of energy lately or full of exciting ideas?

Biological symptoms

- How is your sleep?
- Do you need less sleep than usual?
- How has your appetite been recently?
- Have you lost/gained any weight?

Cognitive symptoms

- How has your concentration been recently?
- Are you able to think clearly?
- Do your thoughts drift off so that you do not take things in?
- Do you find that many thoughts race through your mind?

Eliciting grandiose ideas and delusions

- How do you see yourself compared with others?
- Are you specially chosen in some way?

- Do you have any special powers or abilities quite out of the ordinary?
- Is there a special mission to your life?
- Are you a prominent person or related to someone prominent like the royalty?
- Are you very rich or famous?
- Have you felt especially healthy?
- Have you developed new interests lately?
- Have you been buying interesting things recently?
- Tell me about your plans for the future? Do you have any special plans?

Other issues

- Explore in detail the symptom history, mode of onset, duration, progress, precipitating factor and associated problems
- Rule out co-morbidity such as:
  - Depression
  - Psychotic symptoms
  - Coping mechanisms, i.e., drug and alcohol misuse.

Eliciting hallucinations

TASK: Elicit different types of hallucinations

Auditory hallucinations

- I understand that recently you have been hearing voices when there is no one around you and nothing else to explain it. Can you tell me more about it?

OR

- I should like to ask you a routine question, which we ask of everybody. Do you ever seem to hear voices or noises when there is no one about and nothing else to explain it?

If the patient says 'yes' explore more about it.

Elementary hallucinations

- Do you hear noises like tapping or music?
- What is it like?
- Can you make out the words?
- Does it sound like muttering or whispering?

Second person auditory hallucinations

- Do you hear voices?
- How many voices do you hear?
- Can you give me an example?
- Do they speak directly to you?
- Do they tell you what to do?
- Can you carry on two-way conversion with the voices?
- Do you hear your name being called?
- Who is it you are talking to?
- What is the explanation?

Third person hallucinations

- Do you hear several voices talking about you?

OR

- Do they refer to you as 'he' or 'she' like a third person?
- What do they say?
- Do you hear voices like a running commentary instructing you to do things?
- Do they seem to comment on what you are thinking, reading or doing?
- Do the voices belong to men, women or children?
- Can you recognize those voices?
- If you recognize them, whose voices are they?

Confirm whether they are true hallucinations

- Where do these voices come from?
- Do you hear them in your mind or in your ears?
- Do the voices come from inside or outside your head?
- Do you hear them as clearly as you hear me?
- Can you start or stop them?
- Do you feel that they are real or do you feel that they are just voices?

Hypnagogic/hypnapompic hallucination

- Do these voices disturb your sleep?
- Do you hear them more at any particular time of the day?

Visual hallucination

- Have you seen things that other people can't see?
  - With your eyes or in your mind?
- What did you see?
- Were you half asleep at that time?
- Has it occurred when you are fully awake?
- Did you realize that you were fully awake?
- How do you explain it?

Olfactory hallucination

- Is there anything unusual about the way things feel, taste or smell?
- Do you sometimes notice strange smells that other people don't notice?

Gustatory hallucination

- Have you noticed that food or drink seems to have an unusual taste recently?

Tactile hallucination

- Have you had any strange or unusual feelings in your body?
- Do you ever feel that someone is touching you, but when you look there is nobody there?

Somatic hallucination

- Some people have funny sensations on the body, for example, insects crawling or electricity passing or muscles being stretched or squeezed—have you had any such experiences?
- How do you explain it?

Duration, course, effects, coping

- How long have you experienced them?
- How often do you experience them?
- What do you think might have caused this?
- Why do you think they are happening to you?
- How is it affecting your life?
- How do you manage to cope?
- Do you get any help?

Eliciting delusions and abnormal experiences

TASK: Elicit different types of delusions and other abnormal experiences

Start with open questions and then proceed to closed questions.

- Have you experienced anything strange, bizarre or unusual? Or perhaps something that has puzzled you?
- Does anything interfere with your thoughts in any way?

Delusions of persecution

- How well have you been getting on with people?
- Do you ever feel uncomfortable as if people are watching you or talking about you behind your back?
- Is anyone trying to harm, or interfere with you or make your life miserable?
- Is anyone deliberately trying to poison you or to kill you?
- Is there any organization, such as the Mafia, behind it?

Delusions of reference

- Do people seem to drop hints about you or say things with a special meaning?
- Does everyone seem to gossip about you? Or spy on you?
- Do you see any messages for yourself/reference to yourself on TV or radio or in the newspapers?
- Do things seem to be specially arranged?

Delusions of control

- Is anyone trying to control you?
- Do you feel that you are under the control of a person or force other than yourself?
- Do you feel as if you are a robot or zombie with no will of your own?
- Do they force you to think, say or do things?
- Do they change the way you feel in yourself?

Delusions of grandiosity

- How do you see yourself compared with others?
- Is there something out of the ordinary about you?

- Do you have any special power or abilities?
- Are you specially chosen in any way?
- Is there a special mission to your life?
- Are you a prominent person or related to someone prominent like royalty?
- Are you very rich or famous?
- What about special plans?

Delusions of guilt

- Do you feel you have done something wrong?
- Do you have any regrets?
- Do you have guilt feelings as if you have committed a crime or a sin?
- Do you feel you deserve punishment?

Nihilistic delusions

- How do you see the future?
- Do you feel something terrible has happened or will happen to you?
- Do you feel that you have died?
- Has part of your body died or been removed?
- Enquire about being doomed, being a pauper, intestines being blocked etc.

Religious delusions

- Are you especially close to God or Christ?
- Can God communicate with you?

Hypochondriacal delusions

- How is your health?
- Are you concerned that you might have a serious illness?

Delusions of jealousy

- Can you tell me about your relationship?
- Do you feel that your partner reciprocates your loyalty?

If the patient says 'yes' to any of the delusions, then pick up the clues from what the patient says to you.

Assess the degree of conviction, explanation, effects and coping. Also assess their onset (primary/secondary) and their fixity (partial/complete).

Conviction, explanation, effects, coping

- What do you think is causing these experiences?
- Who do you think is causing them?
- Why do they do so?
- And how do they do that?
- How would you explain them?
- Ask how he/she copes with these thoughts, what he/she has done and what he/she intends to do about them.

Onset and fixity

Always check whether the delusion is:

- Primary or secondary
  - How did it come into your mind that this was the explanation?
  - Did it happen suddenly or out of the blue?
  - How did it begin?
- Partial or full
  - Even when you seemed to be most convinced, do you really feel in the back of your mind that it might well not be true, that it might be your imagination?

  OR

  - Do you ever worry that all of this may be due your mind playing tricks?

Eliciting first rank symptoms

TASK: Elicit first rank symptoms of schizophrenia

Schneider's first rank symptoms are:

- Hearing thoughts spoken aloud
- Third person auditory hallucinations
- Running commentary hallucinations
- Thought withdrawal
- Thought insertion
- Thought broadcasting
- Made volition
- Made feelings
- Made impulses
- Somatic passivity
- Delusional perception.

Initial questions

- I gather that you have been through lot of stress and strain recently. When under stress sometimes people have certain unusual experiences. By unusual experience, I mean for example, hearing noises or voices when there is no one around. Have you had any such experiences?

If the patient says 'Yes' explore more about the voices.

- Can you tell me more about the voices?

Third person auditory hallucinations

- Do the voices speak among themselves?
- Do you hear several voices talking about you?
- Do they refer to you as 'he' (or 'she') as a third person?
- What do they say?

Running commentary hallucinations

- Do they seem to comment on what you are thinking, reading or doing?

OR

- Do you hear voices like a running commentary instructing you to do things?

Hearing thoughts spoken aloud

- Can you hear what you are thinking?
- Do the voices repeat your thoughts?
- Do you ever seem to hear your own thoughts echoed or repeated?
- What is it like?
- How do you explain it?
- Where does it come from?

Thought alienation phenomenon (open question)

- Are you able to think clearly?
- Is there any interference with your thoughts?

Thought broadcasting

- Do you feel that your thoughts are private or are they accessible to others in any way?

- Are your thoughts broadcast, so that other people know what you are thinking?
- Can other people read your mind?
- How do you know?
- How do you explain it?

Thought insertion

- Are thoughts put into your head that you know are not your own?
- How do you know they are not your own?
- Where do they come from?

Thought withdrawal

- Do your thoughts ever seem to be taken from your head, as though some external person or force were removing them?

OR

- Do your thoughts disappear or seem to be taken out of your head?
- Could someone take your thoughts out of your head?
- Would that leave your mind empty or blank?
- Can you give an example?
- How do you explain it?

Passivity of feelings or actions

- Are you always in control of what you feel and do?
- Do you feel in control of your thoughts, actions and will?
- Is there something or someone trying to control you?
- Do you feel under the control of some force or power other than yourself, as though you are a robot or a zombie without a will of your own?
- Does this force make your movements for you without you willing it?
- Does this force or power force its feelings onto you against your will?
- Does this force have any other influence on your body?

Somatic passivity

- Are you possessed?
- What does that feel like? How does this force influence you?
- Does it ever make your movements for you?

- Does this force have any other influence on your body?
- Can you describe it for me?

Delusion perception

- Did you at any time realize that things happening around you have a special meaning for you?
- Can you explain that? What happened exactly?

Effects, coping

- What do you think is causing these experiences?
- Who do you think is causing them?
- Why do they do so? And how do they do that?
- How would you explain them?
- Could it be your imagination?
- How long have you had these experiences?
- How do they affect you?
- How do they make you feel?
- How do you cope with them?
- What do you intend to do about them?

Assess insight

TASK: Assess the patient's level of insight

- Do you consider that you are ill in any way?
- Do you have a physical or mental illness?
- Do you think there is anything the matter with you?
- What do you think it is?
- Could it be a nervous condition? What is it?
- Why do you think that you have come into the hospital?
- What do you feel about being in hospital?
- Has the medication been helpful?
- Do you think that medication helps you to remain well?
- Has any other treatment been helpful?
- You described several symptoms, namely (list symptoms). What is your explanation of these experiences?
- Do you think that the symptoms are part of your nervous condition.

Eliciting anxiety symptoms

TASK: Elicit symptoms of anxiety

Anxiety symptoms

- Have there been times when you have been very anxious or frightened?
- What was this like?
- Have you had the feeling that something terrible might happen?
- Do you worry a lot about simple things?
- Have you had the feeling that you are always on the edge?
- Tell me what made you feel so anxious? And tell me about your anxiety symptoms?
- How long have you been feeling so anxious?
- How does it interfere with your life and activities?

Panic attacks

- Have you noticed any changes in your body when you feel anxious?
- Have you had times when you felt shaky, your heart pounded, you felt sweaty and dizzy and you simply had to do something about it?
- Were you getting 'butterflies' in your stomach, 'jelly legs', and trembling of hands?
- What was it like?
- What was happening at the time?
- How often do you get these attacks?
- How does it interfere with your life and activities?

Agoraphobia

- Do you tend to get anxious in certain situations, such as travelling away from home or being alone?
- What about meeting people, for example, in a crowded room?
- What about situations such as being in a lift or tube?
- Do you tend to avoid any of these situations because you know that you'll get anxious?
- How much does it affect your life?

Special phobias

- Do you have any special fears like some people are scared of cats or spiders or birds?

Other issues

- Explore in detail about the symptom history, mode of onset, duration and progression of symptoms
- Rule out co-morbidity
  - Depression
  - Obsessional symptoms
  - Coping mechanisms.

Eliciting obsessive-compulsive symptoms

TASK: Elicit symptoms of obsessive compulsive traits/disorder

Obsessional symptoms

- Do any unpleasant thoughts/ideas keep coming into your mind, even though you try hard not to have them?

OR

- Do you have any recurring thoughts, ideas, or images that you cannot get rid of from your mind?
- Where do they come from?
- Are these thoughts your own or are they put into your mind by some external force?
- What is it like? How do you explain it?
- How often do you have these thoughts?
- What do you do when you get these thoughts?
- Are they distressing and, if so, in what way?
- Is there anything you try to do to stop these thoughts?
- What happens when you try to stop them?

Compulsive symptoms

- Do you find that you have to keep on checking things that you know you have already done, such as gas taps, doors and switches?
- What happens when you try to stop checking them?
- Do you spend a lot of time on personal cleanliness, such as washing over and over even although you know that you are clean?
- Does contamination with germs worry you?
- Do you have to touch or count things many times?
- Do you have any other rituals?

- Do you find it difficult to make decisions even for simple trivial things? (obsessional ruminations)
- Do you have any impulses to do unwise things?
- What kind of things, and do you ever give in to these impulses?

Other issues

- Explore in detail about the symptom history, mode of onset, duration, precipitating factors and associated problems
- Ask about associated symptoms, such as:
  - Depression, generalized anxiety, phobias
  - Anankastic personality traits—do you tend to do things/keep things in an organized way?

Eliciting premorbid personality

TASK: Elicit premorbid personality

Start with open questions:

- How would you describe yourself as a person before you were ill?
- How do you think other people would describe you as a person?

Then ask closed questions about individual personality traits.

Cluster A

- How do you get on with people? (paranoid)
- Do you trust other people? (paranoid)
- Would you describe yourself as a 'loner'? (schizoid)
- Were you able to make friends?
- Do you have any close friends? (schizoid)
- Do you indulge in fantasies—sexual and non-sexual fantasies, daydreaming?
- Do you like to be around other people or do you prefer your own company?

Cluster B

- What's your temper like? (antisocial, emotionally unstable)
- How do you deal with criticism?
- Are you an impulsive person? (impulsive)
- Do you take responsibility for your actions? (antisocial, impulsive)
- Are you over-emotional (histrionic)

Cluster C

- How do you cope with life? (anxious, borderline)
- How do you react to stress? (borderline, anxious)
- Do you maintain long-term relationships with people? (antisocial, borderline)
- Do you often feel that you are empty inside?
- Are you anxious or shy? (anxious, avoidant)
- Are you a worrier? (anxious, dependent)
- How much do you depend on others? (dependent)
- Would you describe yourself as a perfectionist? (anankastic)
- Do you tend to keep things in an orderly way? (anankastic)
- Do you have unusually high standards at work/home? (anankastic)

Other questions

Also ask about:

- Predominant mood
  - Optimistic/pessimistic
  - Stable/prone to anxiety
  - Cheerful/despondent
- Interpersonal relationships
  - Current friendships and relationships
  - Previous relationship—ability to establish and maintain
  - Sociability—family, friends, workmates and superiors
- Coping strategies
  - How does the patient cope with problems?
  - When you find yourself in difficult situations, what do you do to cope?
  - What sort of things do you like to do to relax?
- Personal interests—hobbies, interests
- Beliefs—religious beliefs. Are you religious?
- Habits—food fads, alcohol, current/ previous use of drugs, etc.

Mini mental state examination*

TASK: Carry out mini mental state examination

The points to be covered are:

Temporal orientation, spatial orientation, registration, attention, concentration, recall, naming, repetition, comprehension, reading, writing, copying.

*Modified from Folstein et al. (1975)

Orientation to time

- What is the year? (1 score)
- What is the season? (1 score)
- What is the month? (1 score)
- What is the day of the week? (1 score)
- What is the date? (1 score)

Orientation to place

- What is the country? (1 score)
- What is the county/state/province? (1 score)
- What city are we in? (1 score)
- What is the name of the hospital or building? (1 score)
- What floor are we on? (1 score)

Registration

- Repeat till you remember: apple, table, penny. (3 score)

(The first repetition determines his/her score but keep saying them until he/she can repeat all 3, up to 6 trials)

Attention and concentration

- Spell the word 'WORLD'; now try to spell it backwards D-L-R-O-W. (5 score)

Recall

- What were the three words that you were asked to remember? (3 score)

Naming

- What is this called? (show a watch)
- What is this called? (show a pencil) (2 score)

Repetition

- Repeat after me 'No ifs, ands or buts'. (1 score)

Reading

- Read and do what is written down 'CLOSE YOUR EYES'. (1 score)

Writing

- Write a short sentence. (1 score)

Copying

- Copy this drawing (2 interlocking pentagons). (1 score)

Comprehension

- Take this paper in your right hand, fold it in half and put it on the floor. (3 score)

Bedside tests for cognitive function

TASK: Carry out bedside tests for cognitive function

Attention and concentration

- Serial recitation tasks-Digit span test
- Serial reversal tasks
  - Spelling W-O-R-L-D backwards
  - Reciting months of the year backwards
  - Serial 7s.

Calculations

- Addition
- Subtraction
- Multiplication.

Memory—new learning

- Registration and 3 to 5 minute recall of 3 or 4 words
- Memory phrase—8 items:

  Mr. John Brown,
  42, West Street, Bedford
  England

Repeat until the subject recalls completely correctly, or stop after five repetitions.

Remote memory/long-term memory

- Personal events
  - When did you get married?
  - When did you finish school?
- General events
  - Who is the current prime minister of the UK?
  - Who is the previous prime minister of the UK?
  - Who is the current president of USA?
  - Who is the previous president of USA?
  - What are the years of World War II?
  - Has anything important happened in the world recently—description of any recent news events, e.g., political, sports events, accidents, catastrophes?

Language

- Comprehension—simple commands, e.g., close your eyes, touch your nose
- Repetition—repeat 'No ifs, ands or buts'
- Naming—point to two or three objects and ask the patient to name them. Use readily available items of clothing and furniture including global names (e.g., watch, jacket) and more specific items (e.g., label or winder) that are generally more difficult
- Word fluency—ask patients to generate a list of as many animals as possible in 1 minute (normal: 15 in a category in 1 minute)
- Reading—single words, passages
- Writing—single words and sentences.

Perception and constructions

- Visuospatial
  - Copy intersecting pentagons
  - Copy a triangle.
- Right-left orientation
  - E.g., point to body part on right/left side of the body.
- Hemi-spatial neglect
  - Ask patient to bisect drawn line
- Drawing and copying
  - Draw a circle and ask the subject to fill in numbers and hands to current time and tell the subject what the current time is. This can indicate perceptual and perceptuomotor deficits, constructional apraxia and unilateral neglect.

Praxis

- Combing hair
- Brushing teeth.

Frontal lobe function testing

TASK: Carry out frontal lobe function tests

Frontal executive function tests

- Assessment of verbal fluency
  - Patient is asked to name as many words as possible beginning with either the letters 'F, A or S' (ideally all three ought to be tested) in 1 minute
  - Alternatively, you can use a category (name as many animals as possible in 1 minute)
  - Normal subjects should produce at least 15 words for each letter
- Assessment of abstraction
  - Proverb interpretation—ask the patient the meaning of two common proverbs:
    a. *Example 1:* 'Too many cooks spoil the broth'
    b. *Example 2:* 'A stitch in time saves nine'
  - Similarities—the patient is asked to explain the similarities between things (use things that are routinely used)
    a. *Example 1:* table and chair
    b. *Example 2:* apple and orange
  - Cognitive estimates—how tall is the average man in the UK?
- Coordinated movements (tests response inhibition and set shifting)
  - Alternate sequence—an alternating sequence is shown to the patient, and they are asked to copy it
  - Go/no-go test—ask the patient to place a hand on the table and to raise one finger in response to a single tap, while holding still in response to two taps. You tap on the undersurface of the table to avoid giving visual cues
  - Luria three-step task—a sequence of hand positions is demonstrated (fist-edge-palm) five times and the patient is asked to repeat it.
- Primitive reflexes: check for primitive reflexes such as grasp reflex, pout reflex and palmomental reflex.

5

Aetiological formulation

Every candidate in part 2 is expected to be able to address the question:

'Why has this patient developed this disorder at this point in their life?'

Remember the 3 Ps:

- **Predisposing** factors
- **Precipitating** factors
- **Perpetuating** factors.

Consider biological, psychological and social causes and cross-tabulate these with predisposing, precipitating and perpetuating factors (see Table 5.1)

Candidates are not expected to 'fill in' every one of the boxes in Table 5.1, but you will have had to think about each.

For an example using schizophrenia see Table 5.2.

TABLE 5.1 Structure of an aetiological formulation

Aetiological factors	Biological factors	Psychological factors	Social factors
Predisposing			
Precipitating			
Perpetuating			

TABLE 5.2 Example of a dimensional approach to the aetiology of schizophrenia

Aetiological factors	Biological factors	Psychological factors	Social factors
Predisposing	Genetic risk	Schizotypal personality	Urban birth
Precipitating	Cannabis misuse	High expressed emotion	Life events
Perpetuating	Non-compliance with treatment	Poor insight	Homelessness

Aetiology

Commonly identified aetiological factors

- Recent stressful life events
- Noncompliance with medications
- Non-engagement with services
- Lack of insight
- Substance misuse
- Co-morbid physical illnesses
- Social isolation
- Poor financial support, lack of employment, housing
- Poor premorbid adjustments
- Previous history of mental illness
- Family history of mental illness
- Recent bereavement (elderly)
- Sensory deprivation (elderly).

The other aetiological risk factors specifically to be looked for in the common psychiatric conditions given are outlined below.

Schizophrenia

- Genetic risk—positive family history.

Environmental insults in early development

- Perinatal trauma—obstetric complications
- Perinatal infection—prenatal exposure to influenza
- Urban settings—city birth
- Degree of urbanization at birth.

Childhood period

- Delayed motor developmental milestones, including delayed walking
- Preference for solitary play
- Lower educational test scores at different levels such as age 8, 11 and 15 years
- Low premorbid IQ.

Others

- Children of migrants
- Substance abuse—heavy cannabis intake

- Recent stressful life events
- High expressed emotion (emotional over-involvement, critical comments and hostility)
- City/rural areas.

Depression

Childhood

- Genetic risk
- Parental loss
- Emotional, physical or sexual abuse
- Perceived lack of parental warmth, acceptance and affection
- Disturbed family environment.

Adolescence

- Early onset anxiety disorder
- Early onset conduct disorder
- Presence of neurotic personality traits
- Low self-esteem
- Low educational attainment.

Adulthood

- Stressful life events and ongoing psychosocial stressors
- Poor social support
- Personal history of mood disorder
- Marital problems
- Physical illness
- Substance abuse, e.g., alcohol
- Non-compliance with medication
- Unemployment
- Loss of role
- Negative cognitive style—learned helplessness and Beck's negative cognitive triad
- Lack of perceived control over future
- Positive family history
- Personality—obsessional, dependent, anxious and borderline traits in the personality.

Brown and Harris vulnerability factors

- Having three children under 14 years of age at home
- Lack of paid employment
- Lack of a confidant relationship.

Mania

- Family history
- Non-compliance with medication
- Intercurrent substance misuse
- Recent life event
- Social rhythm disruption—new shift work, recent delivery of a baby, sleep deprivation secondary to long haul flights.

Anorexia nervosa

Predisposing factors

- Personal events—emotional, physical and sexual childhood abuse
- Vulnerable personality—obsessional and impulsive borderline traits in the personality
- Family conflict—enmeshment, over-involvement, scapegoat
- Any psychiatric disorder (depression, anxiety, deliberate self-harm) in the patient
- Positive family history of affective disorder
- Stressful life events
- Social factors—Western society and cult of thinness
- Genetic constitutional—whether vulnerable to weight loss or disordered 5-hydroxytryptamine (serotonin) system
- Early life experiences—parental loss and separation
- Personality traits.

Precipitating factors

- Recent stressful life events
- Treatment issues—recent alteration in drugs or therapies.

Perpetuating factors

- Personality issues
- Family factors
- Primary or secondary gain.

Alcoholism

- Male sex
- Occupation—journalists, doctors, vets, publicans
- Early drinking, life-long
- Positive family history of alcoholism or depression
- Childhood abuse or neglect
- Co-morbid drug misuse
- Previous periods of inpatient or outpatient detoxification
- Relationship and work difficulties
- Forensic history
- Antisocial personality traits/disorder
- Conduct disorder during childhood
- Impulsivity, angry and aggressive personality traits
- Psychiatric history of anxiety, social phobia and depression.

Post-traumatic stress disorder

- Female sex
- Afro-Caribbean/Hispanic
- Lower socioeconomic class
- Lower education
- Presence of neurotic traits
- Presence of low self-esteem
- History of previous traumatic events or childhood experiences
- Past history of mood disorders/anxiety disorders
- Family history of mood disorders/anxiety disorder.

Alzheimer's dementia

- Older age
- Female gender
- Positive family history
- Past history of head injury
- Low educational status
- Down's syndrome

Vascular dementia

- Older age
- Female gender

- History of diabetes mellitus
- History of hypertension and other vascular disease
- Atrial fibrillation
- History of depression
- Cigarette smoking

6

Investigations

Types of investigation

- Physical/medical
- Psychological
- Social.

Physical investigations

Note: do not mention everything in the exam:

- Think, in advance, which investigations are appropriate for your case
- Use your common sense
- Mention the investigations that you carry out in your routine day-to-day practice and those that are appropriate and relevant to your case.

Blood

- Full blood count (FBC)
- B12 and folate levels
- Liver function tests (LFTs)
- Urea and electrolytes (U&Es)
- Creatinine
- Thyroid function tests (TFT)
- Blood sugar.

Where there is suspicion of drug or alcohol dependency, check mean corpuscular volume (MCV), and toxicology screening may be added.

Special tests for selected cases should only be carried out if the history and physical examination warrants it. These tests include:

- VDRL (Venereal Disease Research Laboratory)
- Hepatitis B, hepatitis C
- HIV testing (Human Immunodeficiency Virus).

Urine

- Urine drug screen
- Mid-stream urine—microscopy, culture and sensitivity in elderly patients and where history suggests.

Imaging

- Chest X-ray (CXR)—elderly patients, and only where examination and history suggests morbid respiratory and cardiovascular conditions
- Electrocardiogram (ECG)—only for specific cases (elderly patients and for patients on high dose antipsychotics, special populations with cardiac problems)
- Electroencephalogram (EEG)—requires justification on the grounds of diagnostic need
- Computed tomography (CT)—requires justification on the grounds of diagnostic need
- Magnetic resonance imaging (MRI)—only for specific cases
- Other investigations as dictated by findings on physical examination.

Psychological investigations

- Consider psychometric testing/neuropsychological assessment if you suspect dementia, cognitive impairment, organic psychiatric illness or learning disability
- Rating scales to establish baselines (mood rating scales, anxiety and depression rating scales)
- Personality assessment (only for specific cases)
- Assessment by an educational psychologist for children.

The following types of self-monitoring can be requested if appropriate:

- Mood diary
- Eating or drinking diary
- Activities diary.

Social investigations

Different sources of information include:

- Collateral history from:
  - Partners
  - Relatives
  - Friends
  - Carers (formal and informal) with the *patient's consent*
- Liaising with:
  - GP and primary care staff, e.g., the district nurse
  - Nursing team involved in the patient's care and in the unit
  - Other members of the multidisciplinary team, such as the community psychiatric nurse, social worker, occupational therapist and other professionals
- Notes
  - Previous medical notes/psychiatric notes
  - Nursing notes
  - Previous discharge summaries
  - Care programme approach (CPA) forms and old written care plans
- Reports
  - Occupational therapists assessment report
  - Social workers assessment report
  - Community psychiatric nurses/Care-coordinators report
  - Other relevant report
  - School reports (child and learning disability cases)
  - Court report
  - Police reports
  - Forensic reports.

7

Management

At this point in the exam, you are trying to be an equal colleague of the examiners. You are expected to come across as a specialist registrar (SpR) with whom they would readily leave the ward and the team while they are away.

As part of your examination preparation, you should write out typical structured management plans for common conditions, such as schizophrenia, affective disorders, neurotic disorders, substance misuse, eating disorders and older age psychiatric disorders.

The management plan should be tailored according to the individual case that you see on the day of the exam.

Management plan

The management plan should be divided into:

- Immediate/short term management
- Long-term management.

Remember:

- 'Biopsychosocial model' (physical, psychological and social)
  - Psychopharmacological treatment
  - Psychotherapeutic interventions
  - Psychosocial interventions
- Multidisciplinary team approach.

Immediate/short-term management

Medical management

Psychopharmacological/physical

- Medication (antipsychotics, antidepressants, mood stabilizers, benzo-diazepines and medications for physical health problems)—discussed in detail in the latter part of this book
- Electroconvulsive therapy (ECT)—if appropriate.

Nursing

Nursing assessment involving:

- Observation of behaviour
- Monitoring of biological functions, such as sleep pattern and appetite
- Checking compliance with medication and personal hygiene
- Providing emotional and practical support (if necessary in the unit)
- Encouraging the patient to attend ward activities
- Different levels of observation according to the patient's current mental state
- Referral to day hospital
- Routine urine and drug screening for selected cases.
- Comprehensive risk assessment.

Psychological management

Please mention the following only if appropriate to your case.

- Advice and structured counselling
- Psychoeducation for the patient and the family
- Compliance therapy
- Insight-oriented therapy
- Supportive psychotherapy
- Behaviour therapy (child psychiatry, learning disability and selected cases)
- Drug education/ motivational programme (drug and alcohol misuse)
- Involve the psychologist to identify and develop successful coping strategies for both the patient and the relatives and to identify the mode of psychological support that patients may require on a long-term basis, including:
  - Cognitive behavioural therapy (CBT)—individual and group
  - Family therapy assessment
  - Psychodynamic—individual, group therapy assessment
  - Cognitive analytical therapy (CAT)
  - Dialectical behavioural therapy (DBT).

Social

- Involve *occupational therapists* to carry out occupational therapy assessments including home assessments:
  - To determine activities of daily living (ADL) skills, level of functioning and to ascertain the level of support needed
  - To enhance their life skills training, social skills training, problem-solving skills and relaxation techniques
  - To focus on rehabilitation, mainly vocational rehabilitation, to regain their lost skills and to build up their confidence
- Involve a *social worker and social services* who could help with:
  - Community care assessment and assessment of needs
  - Support regarding placement, benefits, employment and leisure activities
  - In elderly patients—will determine the need for homecare provision such as a home carer, 'meals-on-wheels', financial support, day centre attendance and respite care, and for long-term placement
- Involve *community psychiatric nurses* (CPNs):
  - To monitor the mental state in the community, compliance with medications, efficacy and tolerability of medications
  - To provide additional support such as anxiety management, stress management, relaxation training and relapse prevention work
  - To identify early-relapse indicators
  - Can key work or care coordinate involve various agencies?
- Predischarge care programme approach (CPA) meetings and care plan.

Legal

- Section/guardianship order/supervised discharge
- Court orders
- Police.

Discharge with adequate community support.

Long-term management

The long-term management would focus on:

- Relapse prevention
- Rehabilitation
- Quality-of-life improvement.

Biological

Pneumonic—4Cs:

- *Continue* medications—maintenance therapy and out patient follow-up
- *Community psychiatric nurse* or care-coordinator monitoring in the community
- *Crisis and contingency* plans—assertive outreach team, 24-hour crisis access team
- *Care programme approach*—regular reviews, care plan still in place.

Psychological

- Individual and group CBT
- Family therapy
- Individual/group psychotherapy
- Attendance at day hospital.

Relapse prevention strategies include identifying early warning signs to prevent, identify and intervene for possible precipitant and identifying care pathways.

Social

Pneumonic—8S's:

- **S**elf-help manuals
- **S**elf-help groups
- **S**upport groups
- **S**upport through day centres/drop-ins
- **S**upported education
- **S**upported employment
- **S**upported housing—other placements include independent flats, warden-controlled shelter accommodation, sheltered-plus accommodation, residential placement, residential elderly mentally infirm (EMI) placement, nursing home placement
- **S**ervice interventions—to be increased, such as increased contact with key workers, and improved liaison with primary care services
- Voluntary agencies
- Patient advocacy services.

Schizophrenia

First episode schizophrenia

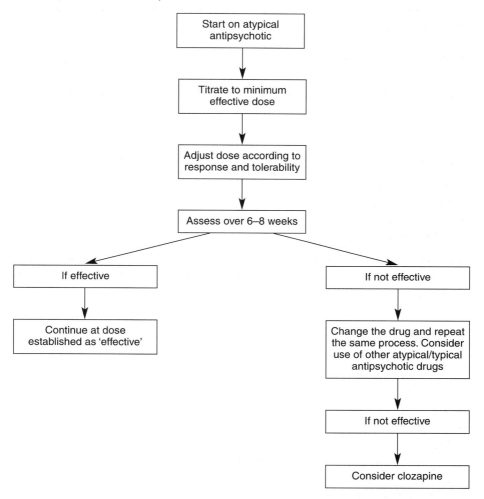

FIGURE 7.1

First episode patients:

- The treatment should focus on bringing *acute symptoms under control* and establishing a long-range treatment plan
- For first episode patients, dosage recommendations tend to be considerably *lower* but some patients may require higher doses than recommended

- Some degree of response is expected within the first *1 to 2 weeks* though the ultimate degree of response can take considerably longer. As a general rule, some clinically significant improvement should be observed within the *first 2 weeks,* and up to 50% of the ultimate improvement may be seen within 4 weeks
- If a reasonable degree of improvement is observed, the following steps should be taken:
  1. Management of adverse effects, if any
  2. Initiation and planning of appropriate psychosocial and rehabilitative services
  3. Family psychoeducation
  4. Implementation of successful follow-up care
- The maintenance treatment is recommended for *1 to 2 years* following a first episode
- For patients presenting with a first episode psychosis, *substance abuse* is an important differential diagnosis to be considered and *urine-screening* tests should be conducted routinely
- *First episode schizophrenia outcome*—87% achieve remission at median period of 11 weeks.

Relapse rates

- Relapse (Lieberman et al, 1996; Robinson et al, 1999):
  - 16% by year 1
  - 54% by year 2
  - 82% by year 5
- After each relapse, 1 in 6 did not remit
- Suicide occurs in 11% of schizophrenic patients
- Patients in good remission for long periods still have an average relapse rate of 75% within 1 to 2 years of discontinuation of medication
- Research evidence also suggests that approximately 16–20% of patients will relapse during the course of a year with adequate pharmacological treatment
- When non-compliance is an additional factor, then as many as 40–50% of patients may experience a relapse within a year
- The abrupt discontinuation of antipsychotics leads to a cumulative relapse rate of 46% at 6 months and 56% at 2 years.

Maintenance treatment

- Following recovery from a first episode of psychosis associated with a schizophrenic illness, *1 to 2 years* is usually the recommendation and the patient should be maintained on a *standard dose of antipsychotic medication*

- For multi-episode patients, these recommendations do not generally exceed 5 years
- If further deterioration of functional capacity occurs with each episode, the recommendations are recommended towards *longer intervals* of maintenance treatment
- Meta-analytic studies of six double-blind randomized controlled trails of low-dose antipsychotic maintenance indicated that *low dose therapy* is not as effective as a *standard dose* in preventing relapse (Barbui et al, 1996)
- Randomized controlled trials on high-dose antipsychotics did not show any significant advantage over a standard dose
- For patients with history of non-compliance, the use of depot drugs should be considered as this can enhance compliance.

Inadequate response to antipsychotics

The following steps should be taken:

- Consider adherence issues and check the *compliance* by *measuring the blood levels* (if possible), which helps to not only confirm the degree of compliance but also to identify individuals with unusually low blood levels despite adequate dosage
- Review the psychiatric *diagnosis*
- Review the *past treatment*
- Rule out *substance abuse*
- Rule out *co-morbidity*, such as affective disorder
- Identify *psychosocial stressors*, to reduce them and help the patient to cope with them.

Next steps:

- Wait in the hope that the patient is slow to respond (questionable)
- Increase the *dose*
- Switching to a *different antipsychotic agent*
- Adding *adjunctive pharmacological* treatment.

If the adherence is doubtful or known to be poor, then investigate the reasons for it.

If the patient is *confused* or *disorganized*, then:

- Simplify the drug regimen
- Consider compliance aids
- Reduce the anticholinergic dosage as it can worsen the confusion.

If the patient lacks *adequate insight*, then consider:

- Compliance therapy
- Depot antipsychotic.

If the patient does not seem to *tolerate* then:
- Discuss with the patient
- Consider switch to acceptable drug with lesser side effects.

Treatment-resistant schizophrenia

Less restrictive definition of treatment-resistant schizophrenia (TRS):

> Lack of a satisfactory clinical improvement despite the sequential use of the recommended doses for 6 to 8 weeks of at least two antipsychotic drugs at least one of which should be an atypical.
>
> (NICE, 2002)

Pharmacological strategies

Antipsychotic drugs:

- Ensure adequate trial of atypical antipsychotics (recommended dosage for adequate duration e.g., 6 to 8 weeks)
- Switch to another class of antipsychotic—either second generation atypical or first generation typical antipsychotics: If a patient has been on a conventional agent, and there is reason to switch then a *new generation antipsychotic* should be considered. The choice of drug and dosage will also be influenced by an evaluation of *past treatment response*. If a patient has a history of responding well to a particular agent then *that medication should be considered a first choice* unless other factors come into play
- If all these measures fail, then consider clozapine.

Clozapine:

- *Clozapine* is not recommended unless patients have failed on two other antipsychotic drugs
- The average dose recommended is approximately 450 mg/day but the response is usually seen in the range 150–900 mg/day
- Plasma levels above a threshold of *350–400 ng/ml* are associated with the highest likelihood of response and a duration of *3 to 6 months* trial should achieve some clinically significant improvement in psychopathology
- An adequate trial of 6 to 12 months should be done with clozapine, and the evidence suggests an advantage to longer treatment with clozapine

- Research evidence suggests that clozapine seemed to:
  - Have specific positive effects on hostility, aggression, disorganization and affective symptoms in schizoaffective disorder
  - Improve cognitive functions, such as attention and verbal fluency
  - Reduce the rate of suicidality
  - Reduce the rate of smoking
  - Reduce rates of *relapse* and *rehospitalization*.

Clozapine augmentation—suggested options:

- Amisulpride augmentation (400–800 mg/day)
- Add sulpiride (400 mg/day)
- Add risperidone (2 mg/day)
- Add lamotrigine (25–300 mg/day)
- Add omega 3-triglycerides (2–3 g EPA daily)
- Lithium augmentation.

Other adjunctive treatments:

- Mood stabilizers or anticonvulsants such as *sodium valproate* and *carbamazepine* are used more frequently than lithium for patients with impulsivity, excitement and aggressive behaviour, and they are more likely to improve with these drugs
- *Carbamazepine* is a potent inducer of hepatic enzymes and concomitant administration can cause a 50% or greater reduction in blood levels of antipsychotics medications
- *Antidepressants,* such as selective serotonin (5-hydroxytryptamine) reuptake inhibitors (SSRIs) and tricyclic antidepressants have been widely used as adjunctive treatments but primarily to treat co-morbid depression or post-psychotic depression
- *ECT* is another adjunctive treatment, and it can be effective as an adjunct to clozapine in treatment refractory patients
- The *benzodiazepines* are used to treat agitation, anxiety and irritability. The therapeutic effects develop rapidly but the positive effects are modest, transient and also diminish after a few weeks.

Negative symptoms

The treatment of negative symptoms is a major challenge that most clinicians are facing. *'True flat affect'* is seen in individuals with negative symptoms but not in the case of depression.

Other conditions that may mimic negative symptoms are:

- Depression
- Antipsychotic drug-induced parkinsonian side effects
- Effects of chronic institutionalization
- Withdrawal in response to a frightening psychotic experience.

The pharmacological strategies for the treatment of negative symptoms include:

- Dopaminergic agents: levodopa, amphetamine, bromocriptine mesilate
- Serotonergic agents: fluoxetine hydrochloride, fluvoxamine malate
- Noradrenergic agents: propranalol hydrochloride, clonidine
- Glutaminergic agents: cycloserine, glycine.

Cognitive symptoms

The new generation antipsychotic medications can *improve cognitive functioning* to a measurable and statistically significant effect.

- Clozapine has been associated with improvements in *executive function*, *verbal fluency*, and *fine motor function*
- Risperidone has been associated with improvement in *attention* and *executive functions*.

Side effects of medications

Typical antipsychotics

- Sedation, dizziness, postural hypotension
- Anticholinergic side effects, such as dry mouth, constipation, blurred vision, urinary retention and confusion in the elderly
- Endocrine effects, including increased appetite, weight gain, diminished libido, impaired ejaculation, amenorrhea, galactorrhoea
- Extra-pyramidal side effects, such as akathisia, acute dystonia, parkinsonism, tardive dyskinesia.

Atypical antipsychotics

- *Olanzapine*—sedation, weight gain, dizziness, postural hypotension, peripheral oedema, anticholinergic side effects such as dry mouth, constipation, hypotension, impaired glucose tolerance and asymptomatic increase in liver enzymes
- *Risperidone*—insomnia, agitation, anxiety, headache, extra pyramidal side effects, postural hypotension especially at the beginning of the treatment, drowsiness, dizziness, nausea, abdominal pain, weight gain, sexual disturbances

- *Quetiapine fumarate*—dizziness, drowsiness, dyspepsia, postural hypotension, weight gain, constipation, dry mouth, hypertension, tachycardia
- *Amisulpride*—insomnia, anxiety, agitation, anticholinergic side effects such as constipation, dry mouth, increased prolactin levels causing amenorrhea, galactorrhoea, loss of libido, breast engorgement
- *Clozapine*—sedation, constipation, dizziness, postural hypotension, transient tachycardia, hyperthermia (fever), hypertension, weight gain, hyper salivation, neutropenia/agranulocytosis, seizures
- *Aripiprazole*—constipation, akathisia, headache, nausea, vomiting, stomach upset, agitation, anxiety, insomnia, sleepiness, lightheadedness, tremor
- *Zotepine*—dry mouth, constipation, dyspepsia, tachycardia, headache, agitation, anxiety, QT interval prolongation, weight gain, sexual dysfunction.

Dosage ranges are given for a number of drugs in Tables 7.1 and 7.2.

TABLE 7.1 Dosage ranges for antipsychotic and other drugs

Drug names	Usual daily dose range (mg)
Typical antipsychotics	
Chlorpromazine	50–1000
Haloperidol	1–20
Trifluoperazine	5–30
Flupenthixol	6–18
Zuclopenthixol	20–150
Sulpiride	200–2400
Atypical antipsychotics	
Olanzapine	5–20
Risperidone	2–8
Quetiapine fumarate	300–750
Clozapine	200–450
Amisulpride	50–300 (negative symptoms)
	400–1200 (positive symptoms)
Zotepine	150–450
Ziprasidone	80–160
Dopamine stabilizer	
Aripiprazole	5–30
Depot medications	
Zuclopenthixol acetate	50–150; IM every 2–3 days
Fluphenazine decanoate	12.5–100; IM every 2 weeks
Flupenthixol decanoate	20–400; IM every 2–4 weeks
Haloperidol decanoate	50–300; IM every 4 weeks
Zuclopenthixol decanoate	200–400; IM every 2–4 weeks
Pipothiazine decanoate	50–200; IM every 4 weeks
Risperidone long-acting injection	25–50; every 2 weeks

TABLE 7.2   Dosage recommendations for newer antipsychotics

Drug	First episode (mg)	Multiple episode (mg)
Olanzapine	5–10	10–20
Risperidone	2–4	4–10
Quetiapine fumarate	200–400	400–750
Amisulpride	30–400	400–1200
Clozapine	100–200	400–900

Advantages of newer atypicals over typical antipsychotics

- Lower propensity to cause extra-pyramidal side effects
- Lower risk of tardive dyskinesia
- Superior efficacy against negative symptoms, depressive symptoms and cognitive symptoms.

As a result of these factors, there could be:

- Enhancement of quality of life
- Improved rates of compliance
- Improved functioning as well as a greater likelihood of participating in psychosocial and vocational therapies.

Management of adverse effects

- Sedation
  - Giving medication all or largely at night can be helpful
  - Dose reduction or changing to a less sedating medication are alternative strategies
- Orthostatic hypotension
  - Gradual dosage escalation can be helpful
  - The patient should be instructed to rise slowly from a seated or prone position
  - Switching to another medication is also helpful
- Extrapyramidal side effects
  - Reduction in dosage
  - Switching to another antipsychotic agent, e.g., olanzapine, quetiapine fumarate, clozapine
  - Use of anticholinergic agents, such as procyclidine hydrochloride, orphenadrine, biperiden, trihexyphenidyl hydrochloride
  - Acute dystonic reaction—intramuscular medication, either anticholinergic or antihistaminic
- Akathisia
  - Reduce the dose or slow down the increase of potential causative agent

- Consider use of lower potency agents
- Beta-blocker such as propranolol hydrochloride may be helpful
- Benzodiazepines such as clonazepam, diazepam and lorazepam can also be helpful
- Tardive dyskinesia
  - The incidence of tardive dyskinesia was approximately 5% per year of drug exposure with relatively consistent risk occurring for the first 8 to 10 years of treatment
  - The risk has been shown to be five times higher in elderly patients treated with conventional antipsychotic drugs
  - Drug discontinuation or switching to a different medication (atypical antipsychotics) can be helpful
- Weight gain
  - Moderate physical exercise
  - Encourage healthy diet, avoiding high calorie foods
  - Involve dietician if necessary
  - Use lowest therapeutic dose
  - Introduce medication increases slowly
  - Switch to medications that have less effect on weight gain
  - Use adjunctive pharmacological treatments, such as orlistat, methyl phenidate hydrochloride or sibutramine
- Endocrine effects—hyperprolactinaemia
  - It is reversible upon stopping medication
  - It can be associated with painful breasts, swollen breasts, amenorrhoea and galactorrhoea, predispose women to cardiovascular disease and osteoporosis and, in men, there is reduced steroidogenesis and spermatogenesis and sexual dysfunction
  - Consider reduction in dose if the patient's mental state is stable
  - Newer generation medications tend to have much less effect on prolactin with risperidone being the most likely and quetiapine fumarate and clozapine the least likely to cause prolactin elevation
  - Asymptomatic hyperprolactinaemia in itself does not warrant change to medication
- Sexual dysfunction
  - Erectile dysfunction, ejaculatory disturbances and loss of libido can occur in men and diminished libido and anorgasmia can occur in women with use of antipsychotics
  - Reducing dosages or switching medications is sometimes necessary
  - Consider switching to alternative agents, such as low-dose olanzapine, quetiapine fumarate and clozapine
  - Imipramine has been used for treating retrograde ejaculation

- Yohimbine hydrochloride, cyproheptadine hydrochloride and sildenafil citrate have been helpful for some patients with erectile dysfunction
- Metabolic syndrome
  - Core features:
    a. Obesity—central or upper body
    b. Insulin resistance or hyperinsulinaemia
    c. Dyslipidaemia
    d. Impaired glucose tolerance or type 2 diabetes mellitus
    e. Hypertension
  - Metabolic syndrome is identified more in patients on atypical antipsychotics, but it can occur in patients on typical antipsychotics as well
  - Lifestyle and risk factor modification, such as reduced dietary fat content, increased physical activity, avoid smoking, reduced alcohol intake, monitoring weight, monitoring metabolic markers (e.g., glucose and lipid profile), can reduced the morbidity and mortality rate, improve the level of function and provide a better quality of life.

Issues of non-compliance

Factors contributing to non-compliance in schizophrenia

- Patient-related
  - Lack of insight
  - Lack of education about the illness
  - Symptom severity
  - Denial
  - Delusional beliefs
  - Co-morbid conditions
- Treatment related
  - Medication side effects, particularly extra-pyramidal side effects (EPSEs), weight gain and sexual dysfunction
  - Complex prescribing regimens
- Environmental factors
  - Inadequate social support
  - Stigma.

Compliance aids (e.g., Medidose system)

The ultimate aim should be to promote independent living, perhaps with the patient filling their own compliance aid, having first been given support and training, but the patient should be clearly motivated to adhere to the prescribed treatment.

Psychosocial management strategies

Psychosocial treatment should be provided to patients, families and to significant others involved in their care. The approach should be *tailored* to the special needs of individual patients.

Psycho-education

Individual psycho-education to be offered to the patient regarding:

- The nature of the illness
- The characteristic symptoms of the illness
- Available treatment options
- The therapeutic effects and side effects of medications
- Discussion of the longer treatment plan
- Identifying early warning signs of relapse.

Compliance therapy

This consists of *four to six* sessions based on motivational interviewing and cognitive *psycho-educational* approaches to psychotic symptoms It also emphasizes the importance of the *treatment alliance* and *patient participation*.

Cognitive behavioural therapy

Individual and group therapies employing well-specified combinations of *support, education,* cognitive and behavioural approaches, social-skills training approaches. It also enhances other targeted problems such as *medication non-compliance.* Cognitive behavioural therapy in addition to drug treatment reduces persistent *positive symptoms*.

The cognitive components involve:

- Identifying links between thoughts, emotions and behaviour and identifying automatic thoughts
- Hypothesis testing about abnormal beliefs and reframing attributions
- Identifying and enhancing coping strategies.

The behavioural elements involve:

- Symptom monitoring
- Use of diary
- Distraction techniques, which focus strategies for hallucinatory experiences
- Graded task assignment
- Anxiety management and relaxation techniques.

Family therapy

Family psychosocial interventions usually last for at least 9 months and provide a combination of:

- Education about the illness and its management
- Family support
- Focusing on strategies to reduce stress within the family
- Maintaining reasonable expectations for the patient's performance
- Crisis intervention.

The various approaches commonly focus on positive areas of family functioning and increasing family structure and stability through problem solving, goal setting and cognitive restructuring.

- It should also be offered to non-family caregivers
- It should not be restricted to patients whose families are identified as having high levels of expressed emotion
- The family interventions are known to be effective in reducing relapse.

Other approaches

- *Motivational intervention techniques* can reduce street drug use and enhance treatment compliance
- *Cognitive remediation* in chronic schizophrenia aims to treat patients on specific neuropsychological tasks, and it reduces cognitive deficits in chronic schizophrenia
- *Social skills training* uses learning theory principles to break complex repertoires down into simpler tasks, subjects them to corrective learning and applies them in real life settings, thereby helping the patient to regain and improve social skills
- *Vocational rehabilitation* includes prevocational training, transitional employment, supported employment, vocational counselling and education services (job clubs, rehabilitation counselling, post-employment services).

Other service provision

- *Day hospitals*
  - These can provide an alternative to inpatient care in certain situations
  - It is a semi-residential structure in which short- and medium-term therapeutic and rehabilitative programmes are carried out
  - It is intended for patients with subacute psychiatric disorders who are in need of drug therapy, psychotherapy and/or rehabilitative therapy

- Its purpose is to avoid, as far as possible, the need for a full-time hospital stay during periods of patient relapse or inability to cope, and to limit the duration of such a stay if it becomes a necessity
- *Assertive community treatment programmes* should be targeted to individuals at high risk for repeated hospitalizations or who have been difficult to retain in active treatment with more traditional types of services
- The *care programme approach* (CPA) plays a major role in:
  - Assessing patient's clinical and other needs
  - Formulating a 'written care plan' with a planned programme of care
  - Identifying a care manager or care coordinator to maintain contact with the patient
  - Arrange discharge planning CPA meeting
  - Coordinate all the members involved in the patient's care
  - Arrange regular reviews once every 6 months with all members involved in the patient's care
- *Community mental health teams* (CMHT) also provide effective treatment with comprehensive assessment of individual patients, provide support and monitor the patient for early warning signs of relapse.

Depression

Mild depression

The treatment involves the following steps:

- *Watchful waiting*—in mild depression, if the patient does not want treatment or may recover with no intervention, arrange for further *assessment,* normally within 2 weeks
- *Sleep and anxiety management*—consider advice on sleep *hygiene* and *anxiety* management
- *Structured and supervised exercise programme*—duration between 10 and 12 weeks, up to 3 sessions per week of moderate duration, each session lasting for 45 minutes to 1 hour
- *Guided self-help*—this consists of provision of appropriate *written materials* and limited support over 6 to 9 weeks, including follow-up from a *professional* who introduces the programme and reviews the progress and outcome
- *Psychological interventions*—the treatment should specifically focus on depression *(brief CBT, problem solving therapy and counselling)* of 6 to 8 weeks over 10 to 12 weeks
- Where significant co-morbidity exists, consider extending treatment duration or specifically focusing on co-morbid problems

- *Antidepressants*—generally not recommended for mild depression, as the *risk-to-benefit ratio* is poor.

However, consider use of an antidepressant for mild depression if:

- It persists after other interventions
- It is associated with medical problems
- It is associated with psychosocial problems
- If a patient with a previous history of moderate or severe depression presents with mild depression.

For patients with depression referred to specialist care, assess patients including their symptom profile, suicide risk, and previous treatment history.

Moderate or severe depression

In moderate depression, offer antidepressant medications to all patients routinely before psychological interventions.

The selection of medications depends on the following factors:

- Severity of the illness
- Previous response to medications
- Response in family members
- Sex of the patient
- Side effect profile
- Toxicity in overdose
- Co-morbidity
- Special features, such as atypical symptoms and psychotic symptoms.

Monitor the risk and review patients periodically.

For patients with a moderate or severe depressive episode, continue antidepressants for *at least 6 to 9 months* after remission.

- SSRIs are recommended as the first line drugs because they are as effective as tricyclic antidepressants and are less likely to be discontinued due to the side effects; tricyclics are more dangerous in overdose (with the exception of lofepramine hydrochloride)
- Consider using a more generic form such as fluoxetine hydrochloride or citalopram as they are associated with fewer discontinuation or withdrawal symptoms.

Once a patient has taken antidepressants for 6 months after remission, review the need for continued antidepressant treatment. This review may include consideration of the number of previous episodes, presence of residual symptoms and concurrent psychosocial difficulties.

- If the patient has not responded well, then check that the drug has been taken regularly and at the prescribed dose
- If the response is inadequate and if there are no significant side effects, consider a gradual increase in dose
- If there is no response after 6 to 8 weeks, consider switching to another antidepressant
- But if there has been a partial response, the decision to switch can be postponed for another 6 weeks.
- If the antidepressant has not been effective, or is poorly tolerated, and the decision is made to offer a further course of antidepressants, then switch to another single antidepressant, such as a different SSRI or mirtazapine, reboxetine or a tricyclic antidepressant
- Inpatient treatment should be considered for people with depression where the patient is at significant risk of suicide or self-harm.

Common causes of hospitalization

- Serious imminent risk of suicide
- Serious long-term high risk of suicide
- Serious risk of harm to others
- Risk of self-neglect
- Severe depressive symptoms
- Severe psychotic symptoms
- Lack of adequate social support
- Severe co-morbid conditions and physical health conditions
- Treatment-resistant cases.

Maintenance therapy

First episode

- The antidepressant treatment should be continued for *6 months to 1 year* after remission, particularly if there are residual symptoms
- The discontinuation should be gradual over a period of *4 to 6 months.*

Recurrent episodes

- Where the depression is chronic or recurrent, assess:
  - Psychosocial stressors
  - Personality factors
  - Significant relationship difficulties

- In co-morbid depression and anxiety, treat the *depression* as a priority
- Continue antidepressant *for 2 years* for people who have had two or more depressive episodes in the recent past and who have experienced functional impairment during the episodes
- To prevent relapse, maintain the antidepressant *at the same dose* at which acute treatment was effective
- Beyond 2 years, for further continuation of the treatment, *re-evaluate* patients on maintenance treatment bearing in mind the patients' age, co-morbid conditions and other risk factors
- If the period between the episodes is less than 3 years or if it is a severe episode, then prophylactic treatment should be maintained for at least 5 years, as the risk of relapse on stopping medication is 70–90% within 5 years.

Refractory depression

Treatment-resistant depression is defined as failure to respond to adequate courses (dose and duration—maximum BNF dose for at least 6 weeks) of two antidepressants or an antidepressant and ECT.

Treatment resistant depression

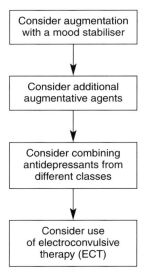

FIGURE 7.2

Treatment strategies

First choice:

- Add lithium (aim for a plasma level of 0.4–0.6 mmol/L)
- Add electroconvulsive therapy
- Add high-dose venlafaxine (>200 mg/day)
- Add triiodothyronine (20–50 µg/day)
- Add tryptophan
- Fluoxetine and olanzapine.

Venlafaxine hydrochloride may be considered for patients who have failed adequate trials of alternative antidepressants. For patients prescribed with venlafaxine hydrochloride, consider monitoring *cardiac function and* undertake monitoring of *blood pressure* for patients on a higher dose.

Consider augmenting an antidepressant with another antidepressant (SSRIs or mirtazapine) and when augmenting one with another, monitor carefully particularly for the symptoms of *'serotonin syndrome'*.

Second choice:

- Add pindolol (5 mg tds)
- Add dexamethasone (4 mg daily for 4/7)
- Add lamotrigine (200 mg/day)
- High-dose tricyclics (imipramine 300 mg/day)
- Add buspirone hydrochloride
- Add monoamine oxidase inhibitors (MAOIs) and tricyclic antidepressant e.g., trimipramine and phenelzine sulphate.

Psychotic depression

- For depression with psychotic features, *ECT should be considered as first line therapy* with significant benefit in 80–90% of cases
- It would be ideal to commence treatment with an *antipsychotic agent* for a few days before commencing an antidepressant, and use of lowest effective dose of antipsychotics is recommended
- When combination treatments of antipsychotic and antidepressants are used, careful dose titration is necessary as it may worsen the side effects common to both
- Following combination treatment, the maintenance often involves a clinically effective antidepressant with the lowest effective antipsychotic dose.

Atypical depression

- Consider prescribing MAOIs such as *phenelzine* for patients whose depression has atypical features, on a dose of 15 mg/day increased gradually to 60–90 mg/day and other MAOIs if necessary; clinically significant advantage in response and remission: Pane et al, 1991 and McGrath et al, 2001
- All patients receiving phenelzine require careful monitoring including *blood pressure* and advice on interaction with other *medicines or foodstuffs*
- Alternatives include SSRIs and the noradrenergic reuptake inhibitor (NARI) reboxetine.

Treatment with electroconvulsive therapy

The selection of ECT may be affected by:

- Patient preference
- Previous recovery with ECT
- Previous experience of ineffective and or intolerable medical treatment.

ECT should only be used:

- To achieve *rapid and short-term* improvement of *severe* symptoms after an adequate trial of other treatments has proven ineffective
- When the condition is considered to be potentially *life-threatening* in a *severe* depressive illness and when the patient is at significant risk of harming themselves or others (potentially life-threatening)
- For a severe depressive episode with severe biological features, such as significant weight loss or loss of appetite
- Where psychotic features are prominent (depressive delusions and or hallucination)
- In patients who are unable to tolerate the side effects of drug treatment
- When there is a previous history of good response to ECT, if used already
- When there is marked psychomotor retardation
- When there is catatonia or stupor
- When there is treatment-resistant psychoses and mania.

Electroconvulsive therapy is not recommended as a maintenance therapy because its longer term benefits and risks have not been clearly established (NICE, 2003).

A repeat course of ECT should be considered under the circumstances indicated above only for individuals who have severe depressive illness and who have *previously responded well* to ECT.

Antidepressants

Side effects

- *Tricyclic antidepressants* (amitriptyline, clomipramine, dothiepin hydrochloride, doxepin hydrochloride, imipramine)—sedation, hypotension, anticholinergic side effects such as dry mouth, constipation, blurred vision, urinary retention, impaired ejaculation, weight gain, ECG changes and arrhythmias
- *Tetracyclic antidepressants* (amoxapine, maprotiline hydrochloride, mianserin hydrochloride)—sedation, drowsiness, dizziness, vivid dreams, dry mouth, constipation, blurred vision, headache, weight gain, tremor
- *Post synaptic 5-hydroxytryptamine (serotonin) receptor blockers and reuptake inhibitors* (trazodone hydrochloride and nefazodone hydrochloride)—nausea, drowsiness, dizziness, postural hypotension, fatigue, headaches, anticholinergic side effects, bradycardia and elevation of hepatic enzymes
- *Irreversible monoamine oxidase inhibitors* (isocarboxazid, phenelzine sulphate, tranylcypromine sulphate)—drowsiness, insomnia, agitation, dizziness, weakness, fatigue, diarrhoea, weight gain, oedema, postural hypotension and anticholinergic side effects
- *Reversible inhibitor of monoamine oxidase type A* (RIMA; moclobemide)—nausea, headache, dizziness, insomnia, anxiety, restlessness, dry mouth, blurred vision, rash
- *Selective serotonin (5-hydroxytryptamine) reuptake inhibitors* (fluoxetine hydrochloride, paroxetine hydrochloride, sertraline hydrochloride, citalopram, escitalopram)
  - Gastrointestinal side effects—nausea, vomiting, dyspepsia, abdominal pain, diarrhoea
  - CNS side effects—headache, sweating, anxiety, agitation, insomnia
  - Sexual dysfunction
- *Selective noradrenalin reuptake inhibitors* (SNRIs; venlafaxine hydrochloride)—nausea, headaches, dry mouth, dizziness, sweating, somnolence, sexual dysfunction, elevation of blood pressure at higher doses
- Noradrenergic/specific serotonergic antidepressants (NaSSAs)
  - Mirtazapine—sedation, drowsiness, dizziness, fatigue, increased appetite, weight gain, dry mouth, constipation
  - Reboxetine—insomnia, sweating, dizziness, dry mouth, constipation, tachycardia, urinary hesitancy
  - Duloxetine hydrochloride—nausea, dryness of mouth, constipation, diarrhoea, vomiting, decreased appetite, dizziness, somnolence, insomnia.

Dosages

Table 7.3 gives the dosage ranges for antidepressants.

TABLE 7.3   Dosage ranges for antidepressants

Drug name	Usual daily dose range (mg)
Amitriptyline	100–150
Clomipramine	100–250
Imipramine	100–300
Lofepramine	140–210
Dothiepin hydrochloride	100–225
Doxepin hydrochloride	100–300
Trazodone hydrochloride	150–600
Nefazodone hydrochloride	300–600
Moclobemide	300–600
Phenelzine	45–90
Fluoxetine hydrochloride	20–60
Fluvoxamine hydrochloride	100–300
Citalopram	20–60
Paroxetine hydrochloride	10–50
Sertraline hydrochloride	50–200
Escitalopram	10–20
Venlafaxine hydrochloride	75–375
Mirtazapine	15–45
Reboxetine	8–12
Duloxetine hydrochloride	60–120

Licensed indications

- Amitriptyline—depression, nocturnal enuresis in children
- Clomipramine—depression, phobic and obsessional states
- Dothiepin hydrochloride, doxepin hydrochloride—depression
- Phenelzine sulphate—depression
- Moclobemide—depression, social phobia
- Trazodone hydrochloride—depression, anxiety
- Nefazodone hydrochloride—depression anxiety
- Fluoxetine hydrochloride—depression, anxiety, obsessive-compulsive disorder (OCD), bulimia nervosa
- Paroxetine hydrochloride—depression, anxiety, OCD, panic disorder, agoraphobia, social phobia, post-traumatic stress disorder (PTSD), generalized anxiety disorder
- Citalopram—depression, anxiety, panic disorder, agoraphobia
- Escitalopram—depression, anxiety, panic disorder, agoraphobia

- Sertraline hydrochloride—depression, anxiety, OCD
- Fluvoxamine malate—depression, OCD
- Venlafaxine hydrochloride—depression, generalized anxiety disorder
- Mirtazapine—depression
- Reboxetine—depression
- Duloxetine—depression.

Psychological treatments

The use of the psychological therapies is influenced by the severity of the episode, patient preferences and local availability.

- Cognitive behavioural therapy (CBT) is the psychological treatment of choice and an adequate course involves 16 to 20 sessions over 6 to 9 months
- Also consider interpersonal therapy (IPT) if the patient expresses a preference for it or if you think that the patient may benefit from it
- When patients have responded to a course of individual CBT or IPT, consider offering follow-up sessions, typically 2 to 4 sessions over 12 months.

Cognitive behavioural therapy

Consider CBT:

- If a patient with moderate or severe depression refuses antidepressant treatment
- For patients who have not made an adequate response/have limited or poor response to other interventions for depression
- For whom avoiding the side effects often associated with antidepressants is a clinical priority or personal preference
- For patients who express a preference for psychological treatments.

Cognitive behavioural therapy in depression

In depression, there is pervasive negative view of the self, the world and the future.

The cognitive part of the CBT includes *identifying, evaluating and modifying* negative automatic thoughts and dysfunctional beliefs.

It involves thought-challenging based on *Socratic questioning,* where these thoughts are challenged constructively by the therapist and alternative explanations are offered, and it aims to reduce the frequency of negative thoughts.

In depression CBT aims to *restructure* the *negative cognitions* that lead to depression *(arbitrary inference, minimization, maximization, selective abstraction, overgeneralization, dichotomous thinking)*.

The behavioural techniques used include:

- *Activity scheduling* with a plan of action aimed at exploring the relationship between activity and mood
- *Mastery and pleasure* tasks focusing on self-monitoring of pleasure and a sense of mastery associated with activities
- *Graded task assignments* breaks goals into achievable subtasks and help patients to achieve success step-by-step and specific experiments to test negative prediction.

Research evidence for CBT in depression:

- Cognitive behavioural therapy is as effective as antidepressant medication in mild-to-moderate depression
- The combination of CBT and antidepressants is not more effective than either treatment alone in mild-to-moderate depression
- The combination of CBT and antidepressants may be more effective than either treatment alone in severe depression
- Relapse rates are lower with CBT than with antidepressants following discontinuation of treatment.

Cognitive behavioural therapy combined with antidepressant medication:

- For patients who present initially with severe depression
- For all patients whose depression is treatment-resistant or chronic
- For patients with treatment-resistant moderate depression who have relapsed while taking or after finishing a course of antidepressants.

Consider the *combination* of antidepressant medication with individual CBT of 16 to 20 sessions over 6 to 9 months.

Interpersonal therapy

- It is a time-limited weekly therapy for depressed patients
- It focuses more on current relationships than on enduring aspects of the personality
- The therapist takes an active role and explores the connections between the onset of the current symptoms and interpersonal problems in four areas— grief, role transitions, interpersonal role disputes and interpersonal deficits
- The therapist will concentrate on strategies specific to one of these problem areas

- The patient is helped to focus on the therapeutic gains and to develop ways of identifying and tackling depressive symptoms.

Bipolar disorder

Hypomania, mania and mixed episode

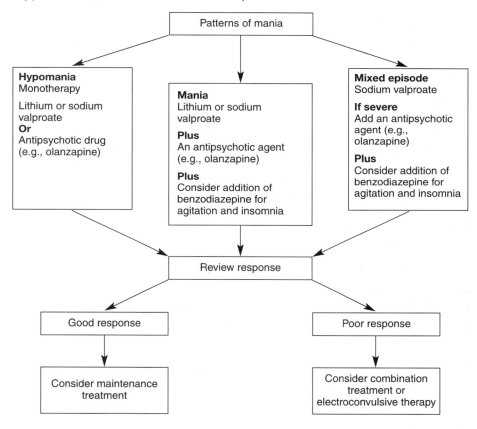

FIGURE 7.3

Key points:

- Antipsychotics, sodium valproate and lithium are *antimanic*. The antipsychotics are preferred in highly active or agitated patients with mania
- The atypical antipsychotics such as olanzapine, risperidone, quetiapine fumarate and aripiprazole have shown *'efficacy as monotherapy'* in placebo controlled trials in mania, and atypicals are less likely to produce extra-pyramidal symptoms

- Short-term treatments of mania can be discontinued after full remission of symptoms, which usually lasts for 2 to 3 months
- If the patient has hypomanic or manic symptoms and if the patient is already on an antidepressant, then *taper and discontinue the antidepressant*
- Just like the switch from mania to depression, a switch from depression to mania can also occur, which may be a consequence either of the *course of the illness or of the treatment*
- If the patient is already on long-term treatment then *'optimize'* and *'continue'* the same treatment
- If the patient is sleep deprived, consider the use of a short-term benzodiazepine. Benzodiazepines are not believed to be antimanic. However, they are used as *adjuncts to other agents* and may be required when sedation or tranquillization is a priority
- The use of benzodiazepines may also reduce the required doses of antipsychotics or other drugs. They should be discontinued after the *desired response* is established
- When on maintenance treatment, if mania recurs, then combining an antipsychotic such as olanzapine, risperidone or haloperidol can facilitate the *acute* treatment response and randomized controlled trials have shown that *combinations are superior to lithium or valproate alone*
- Mixed episodes are *slower* to resolve during treatment than more classic mania.

Depressive episodes

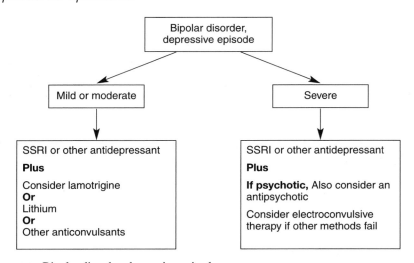

FIGURE 7.4   Bipolar disorder, depressive episode

Key points:

- A switch from mania to depression may occur at any time during the *course of the illness;* it is not established which treatments if any make this more likely to happen
  - If the patient is already on maintenance treatment, then *optimize the therapy and continue*
- Meta analysis has shown that a manic event is *2 to 3 times* more likely to occur during treatment with *tricyclic antidepressants* than during treatment with SSRIs or placebo
- Antidepressants are effective for treating depression in bipolar disorder but are used in combination with an agent that will reduce the risk of mania (lithium, or sodium valproate)
- After remission of an acute episode of depression, the *discontinuation* of antidepressants is currently recommended, but when the risk of a severe depressive episode is high, the antidepressants to which the patient has shown an acute response may be continued long term, either alone or in combination with a drug showing antimanic efficacy
- *Lamotrigine* has been shown to have acute efficacy in depression without a risk of inducing switching
- For manic or mixed states resistant to treatment, or for severe depression *electroconvulsive therapy* provides an important treatment option.

Rapid cycling bipolar disorder

- Taper and discontinue the antidepressants
- Identify and treat factors such as substance misuse, hypothyroidism or lithium-induced hypothyroidism that may contribute
- For initial treatments consider lithium, sodium valproate and lamotrigine— *for rapid cycling disorder, sodium valproate* is the drug of choice
- But, if severe, then add an antipsychotic agent (e.g., olanzapine) and also consider benzodiazepines for agitation and insomnia
- Combinations are often required—evaluate over 6 months or more
- Generally, antidepressant drugs should be stopped and lithium therapy reduced or sometimes stopped in these patients

Maintenance therapy

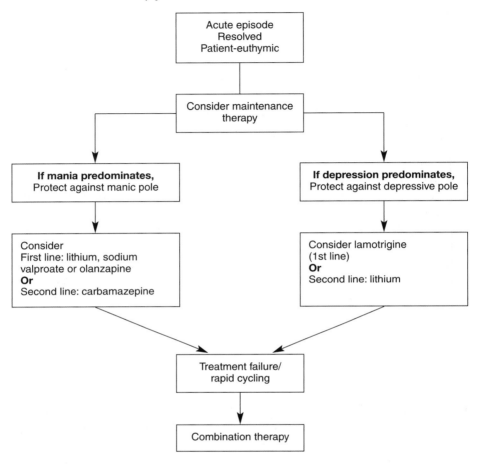

FIGURE 7.5

Key points:

- Lithium and olanzapine prevent the relapse of mania, and research evidence suggests that lithium reduces the risk of *suicide*
- Lithium is probably more effective *against mania* than against depression with a relative risk reduction of *40% and 23%* respectively
- Plasma lithium levels of lithium below 0.5 mmol/L are usually too low to be effective and levels over 0.8 mmol/L are often recommended—the highest dose with the minimal side effects should be employed
- In the prevention of mania, sodium valproate has been proved to be as effective as lithium but carbamazepine is less effective than lithium

- The following conditions predict a relatively poor response to lithium maintenance therapy:
  - Rapid cycling disorders
  - Alcohol and drug misuse
  - Mixed affective states
  - Mood incongruent psychotic features
- Lamotrigine is more effective against depression than mania in long-term treatment, and it has a novel profile in relapse prevention
- Discontinuation of long-term treatment is *not indicated* when there is good clinical control of the illness
- Successful long-term treatment often appears to require *combination* treatment
- Effective prevention of disease progression may require combination therapy from *as early* in the illness course as possible
- Antipsychotic agents may often be appropriate for the long-term management of bipolar patients, especially those in whom *psychotic features are prominent*
- For those who have frequently recurring episodes and either do not benefit from or do not adhere to oral medication, *depot antipsychotic medication* can provide long periods of stability.

Mood stabilizers

Side effects

- *Lithium*—increased thirst, polyuria, polydipsia, bad metallic taste in the mouth, weight gain, nausea, vomiting, abdominal pain, muscular weaknesses, tremors, weight gain, acne, hypothyroidism
- *Carbamazepine*—nausea, vomiting, constipation, sedation (dose-related), dizziness, ataxia, diplopia (dose-related), hepatitis, skin rashes, blood dyscrasias
- *Sodium valproate*—nausea, vomiting, sedation, diarrhoea, ataxia, tremor, hair loss, weight gain, thrombocytopenia, blood dyscrasias, ankle oedema, pancreatitis
- *Lamotrigine*—rash, ataxia, headache, diplopia, vomiting
- *Topiramate*—appetite suppression, weight loss, nausea, abdominal pain
- *Gabapentin*—somnolence, dizziness, ataxia, fatigue.

Dosage

Table 7.4 gives the dosage ranges for mood stabilizers.

TABLE 7.4   Dosage ranges for mood stabilizers

Drug name	Daily dose range recommended (mg)
Lithium carbonate	400–2000
Sodium valproate	500–2500
Carbamazepine	400–1600
Lamotrigine	50–200
Topiramate	25–200

Drug and alcohol misuse

Alcohol dependence

Key features of ICD-10 dependence *(3 items required)* include:

- Compulsion to drink
- Problems in controlled drinking
- Psychological withdrawal symptoms
- Escalating consumption owing to tolerance
- Preoccupation with alcohol to the exclusion of other pursuits
- Increasing time lost to hangovers
- Disregard of evidence that excessive drinking is harmful.

Harmful alcohol use

Harmful use is diagnosed if there is evidence that alcohol is damaging an individual's mental or physical health but the criteria for dependence are not met.

Sensible drinking

- 21 units per week for men
- 14 units per week for women
- people over 65 years of age should consume no more than one standard drink per day, 7 standard drinks per week and no more than 2 drinks at any one time.

Pharmacological management

Detoxification

- Treatment of alcohol use disorders typically involves a combination of pharmacotherapy and psychosocial interventions

- Detoxification is a treatment designed to control both the medical and psychological complications that may occur temporarily after a period of sustained alcohol misuse
- It usually involves chlordiazepoxide at diminishing doses over 7 to 10 days with thiamine supplementation
- The doses of medication should be titrated against withdrawal symptoms.

Outpatient detoxification:

- The benzodiazepines are prescribed in alcohol withdrawal in order to control withdrawal symptoms and to reduce the risk of withdrawal seizures
- Chlordiazepoxide is usually prescribed in a rapidly reducing regimen in order to reduce the development of secondary dependence; it has a lower abuse potential compared with other benzodiazepines
- Chlordiazepoxide is the drug of choice for most uncomplicated alcohol dependent patients, but if there are doubts about compliance or concerns about drinking at any stage during outpatient detoxification, then the patient should be reviewed and breathalyzed before dispensing the next day's supply of the drug.
- Indications for prescribing a reducing regimen:
  - Clinical evidence of alcohol withdrawal features
  - History of alcohol dependence syndrome
  - Consumption of alcohol is greater than 10 units per day over the last 10 days
- Indication for inpatient detoxification:

  - Symptoms of Wernicke-Korsakoff syndrome
  - Past history of seizures or delirium during withdrawals
  - Acute confusional presentation
  - High risk of suicide
  - History of poly drug misuse
  - Co-morbid mental health illness, e.g., depression, psychosis
  - Lack of stable support in the community, e.g., homelessness
  - Severe malnutrition/severe physical health conditions.

Chlordiazepoxide regimen for moderate and severe dependence:

Day 1	20 mg qid
Day 2	15 mg qid
Day 3	10 mg qid
Day 4	5 mg qid
Day 5	5 mg bid

- In severe dependence, even larger doses of chlordiazepoxide may be required and will often require specialist/inpatient treatment

- For inpatient detoxification, the chlordiazepoxide should be prescribed according to a flexible regimen over the first 24 to 48 hours with the dosage titrated according to the severity of withdrawal symptoms. This is followed by a 5-day reducing regimen (a typical regimen might be 10–20 mg qid reducing gradually over 5–7 days). This is usually adequate, and longer treatment is rarely helpful or necessary.

Other medications

- Supplementary vitamins—generally, a 4-week course of 100 mg thiamine tds is recommended, but if there are symptoms suggestive of malnourishment or Wernicke-Korsakoff syndrome then parenteral B vitamins are recommended
- Anticonvulsants—benzodiazepines in sufficient dosage are the most effective anticonvulsant in alcohol withdrawal
- Antipsychotics—it is generally not advisable to start a new psychotropic at this time as most of the antipsychotics reduce seizure threshold. However, if there are psychotic symptoms like delusions or hallucination it could be initially managed by increasing the dose of benzodiazepine. The addition of an antipsychotic, such as haloperidol 5–10 mg orally up to 30 mg/day, should be considered if this fails, but given sufficient benzodiazepine cover you should address the concern of a possible reduction in seizure threshold following antipsychotic use.

Maintenance treatments

Aversive drugs:

- Disulfiram:
  - It is an irreversible inhibitor of acetaldehyde dehydrogenase, which can act as an adjunct to therapy and is prescribed once abstinence is achieved
  - Dose: give a 5-day loading dose of 800 mg/day followed by a maintenance dose of 200 mg or 400 mg on alternate days
  - Common side effects: headache, halitosis
  - Rare reports of hepatotoxicity and psychotic reactions have been reported.

Anti-craving drugs:

- Acamprosate calcium:
  - It is believed to act through enhancing γ-aminobutyric acid (GABA) trans-mission in the brain, and patients taking it report diminished alcohol craving
  - Dose: 666 mg tds, once abstinence is achieved

- Side effects: pruritus, gastrointestinal upset, rash
- Naltrexone hydrochloride:
  - It antagonizes the effects of endogenous endorphins released by alcohol consumption. It appears to be effective in reducing total alcohol consumed and the number of drinking days
  - Dose: 50 mg/day, once abstinence is achieved
  - Side effects: Feeling anxious, headache, fatigue, flu-like symptoms, gastrointestinal symptoms, sleep disturbance.

Research evidence:

- Research has consistently shown that less intensive treatments are as effective as the more intensive options as there was no difference in outcome measures between both groups (Chick et al, 1988)
- Published reports have consistently failed to identify any significant differences in the outcomes between short and long inpatient detoxification programmes (Miller and Hester, 1986)
- Edwards and Guthrie's trial (Edwards and Guthrie, 1967) reported no significant differences in outcomes between the groups who were randomly assigned to inpatient or intensive outpatient treatment and followed up each month for 1 year and assessed by independent raters
- Large trials such as Project MATCH (Matching Alcohol Treatment to Clinical Heterogeneity) and UKATT (The United Kingdom Alcohol Treatment Trial) show no significant difference between the various forms of psychosocial treatment.

Psychosocial intervention

Motivational enhancement therapy

Motivationally based treatments concentrate on strategies that focus on the patient's *own commitment* to change. It combined counselling in the motivational style with objective feedback.

- It is ideal for use in *primary care*
- It is aimed more at the *problem substance misuser* than the dependent substance misuser
- This involves several short sessions of a few minutes aimed at increasing *internal motivation.*

Here, the clients themselves give reasons why they should remain abstinent and draw up a list of problems caused by their alcoholism.

The therapist does not take a directive approach but expresses interest and concern for the patient's problems, uses *open ended questions* and *reflective listening* and aids the *assessment of pros and cons* of current behaviour.

Motivational enhancement therapy also encourages the patient's *own perceptions* of degree of risk, encourages *personal responsibility* and offers patient's a choice of treatment options.

The principles of motivational interviewing—*'FRAMES' formulation:*

F: provide *Feedback* on behaviour
R: emphasis on personal *responsibility* for changing behaviour
A: clear *advice* to change
M: A *Menu* of alternative options to change behaviour
E: therapeutic *empathy* for the patient as a counselling style
S: facilitation of client *self-efficacy* or optimism.

Cognitive behavioural therapy

Cognitive behavioural therapy is now considered to be the most dominant form of psychological intervention for the treatment of substance misuse. It is particularly helpful in co-morbid conditions, such as anxiety disorders, phobic disorders, PTSD, OCD and depression.

Patients who misuse substances are perceived as not having the skills to cope with other problems and this assumes that alcoholism is a maladaptive habit that becomes a means of coping with difficult situations, unpleasant moods and peer pressure.

The emphasis is placed on overcoming *skill deficits* and increasing the *ability to cope* with a difficult situation. One of the main benefits of this approach is to help patients to form the coping strategies and resources to fundamentally prevent relapses.

It is typically offered in the following areas:

- Reducing *exposure* to substances
- *Motivating* by exploring the positive and negative consequences of continued use
- *Self-monitoring* to identify situations, settings, or states associated with higher risk for substance use, and coping with negative emotional states
- *Recognition* of conditioned craving and development of strategies for coping with craving
- *Homework* assignments
- Identification of *thought processes* that can increase risk for relapse, and focusing on relapse prevention
- Social skills training is an integral component of CBT. The techniques include assertiveness training, modelling and role playing of skills such as

refusal of alcohol and dealing with interpersonal problems. It also focuses on dealing with the social pressure to use drugs, development of supportive networks and development of plans to interrupt a relapse.

Twelve-step facilitation

- Twelve-step facilitation is a form of structured intervention to enhance engagement with Alcoholics Anonymous (AA)
- The objectives include encouraging patients to become members of AA groups and to accept the AA philosophy
- The basic philosophy of AA is that of reaching out to other alcoholics to help everyone stay sober
- Group work is central to the approach, and it is grounded in the concept of substance misuse as a spiritual and medical disease.

The *outcomes* for AA attendees are *mixed*, as with all forms of treatment for addiction:

- *Dropout rates are high* and approximately half of those who attend AA leave within 3 months
- Despite this high dropout rate, for those who remain, the abstinence rate is *excellent*; the average length of sobriety amongst active members is *approximately 6 years.*

Brief interventions

Brief interventions are short, focused discussions that usually last less than 15 minutes, which can reduce alcohol consumption in some individuals with hazardous drinking. They are based on motivational interviewing.

These are designed to promote awareness of the negative effects of drinking and to motivate change.

Heterogeneous populations of drinkers in primary care favour screening and brief intervention. A brief intervention involves one or more counselling sessions, which include assessment, motivational work, patient education, comparison of the individual's consumption with drinking norms, feedback about the adverse effects of alcohol, contracting by keeping a drink-diary, setting goals and incentives to reduce weekly consumption and the use of written materials and information leaflets.

Counselling

The patients of all specialist services will benefit from access to formal counselling.

Qualified counsellors who are receiving supervision should deliver formal structured counselling, and professionals who provide counselling will need to ensure that the patient's health and social needs are addressed by different team members. It can address the following:

- Problem-solving skills
- Social skills training
- Anger management
- Relaxation training
- Cognitive restructuring
- Relapse prevention.

Marital and family therapies

Examine the role of important others in the addictive process.

Social behaviour and network therapy

These are focused on improving interpersonal functioning and enhancing social support based on the principle that people with serious drinking problems need to develop a social network that supports change. They use techniques adapted from CBT and help the patients to build these networks.

The patients are encouraged to identify and develop alternative reinforcers, such as fulfilling 'social activities with non-drug using others' and 'vocational rehabilitation'. The provision of constructive and purposeful activity to substitute for the social activity should include educational activities such as attending college and general social activities such as attending social clubs and sport activities.

Practical help

Direct practical help with specific tasks such as physical cleaning of the home, securing housing or making child-care arrangements not only provides some relief, but it also creates a framework of trust within which other therapeutic work may then take place.

Supported accommodation

The provision of housing with 24-hour availability of housing support workers can be of particular assistance in the transition from residential rehabilitation to fully independent living.

Opioid misuse

Opiate withdrawal:

- The withdrawal symptoms appear 6 to 24 hours after the last dose and typically last 5 to 7 days, peaking on the *second or third day*
- Methadone is longer acting and withdrawal symptoms are much more prolonged with symptoms peaking on the *seventh day* or so and lasting up to 14 days.

Pharmacological strategies

Methadone hydrochloride:

- Currently, methadone is the drug of choice used in opiate detoxification regimens and maintenance
- Methadone is a long acting synthetic opioid with a long half-life of 24 hours and is suitable for daily dosing
- It is prescribed as a coloured liquid, available at concentration of 1mg/mL, but it is unsuitable for parenteral use
- At doses of more than 80 mg/day it produces near saturation of opioid receptors, minimizing the reward of further consumption
- Methadone should be initiated according to the severity of withdrawal symptoms—start with 10–20 mg methadone depending on the level of tolerance (low: 10–20 mg; moderate: 25–40 mg)
- Review daily over the first week with dose increments of 5–10 mg/day if indicated; methadone reaches a steady state 5 days after the last dose change
- Stabilization may take *up to 6 weeks to achieve* and during this period the patient should be reviewed regularly after the first week, making subsequent increases by 10 mg on each review up to 120 mg
- In *'rapid reduction regimens'* reduce the dose over 14 to 21 days using symptomatic drugs as adjuncts
- *'Slow reduction'* is to be done gradually *over a period of 4 to 6 months* reducing by 5–10 mg each fortnight
- During the process of reduction regimens, make the largest absolute cuts at the beginning and more gradual cuts as the total dose falls
- Oral methadone is effective in (Welch and Strang, 1999):
  - Reducing illicit drug use
  - Reduced injecting
  - Reduced criminal activity
  - Improved physical health
  - Improved social well-being

- Research evidence has shown that a methadone script reduces street usage, criminality and drug-related mortality.

Buprenorphine (Subutex):

- Buprenorphine is a partial opiate agonist effective in treating opioid dependence.
- It alleviates/prevents opioid withdrawal and craving. It reduces the effects of additional opioid use because of its high receptor affinity.
- It is long-acting and the duration of action is related to the dose administered, and it can be used effectively for shorter-term in-patient detoxifications following the same principles as for methadone.
- Dose increases should be made in increments of 2–4 mg at a time, daily if necessary, up to a maximum daily dose of 32 mg.
- Effective maintenance doses are usually in the range of 12–24 mg daily, which should be achieved within 1–2 weeks of starting Buprenorphine.
- *Lofexidine hydrochloride*
  - Lofexidine hydrochloride is an alpha-adrenergic agonist given as a 7–10 day treatment course, followed by a gradual withdrawal over 2–4 days
  - Start with 200 µg bid, increased in 200–400 µg steps to a maximum of 2.4 mg/day in 2 to 4 divided doses
  - Due to risk of postural hypotension blood pressure should be monitored

Symptomatic medications are used in ameliorating opiate withdrawal symptoms:

- *Metoclopramide hydrochloride*
  - For treatment of symptoms such as nausea, vomiting
  - 10 mg dose up to maximum of 30 mg/day
- *Loperamide hydrochloride*
  - For treatment of diarrhoea
  - 4 mg initial dose with 2 mg after each loose stool, maximum dose 16 mg/day
- *Ibuprofen*
  - For headaches, body aches and muscle pain
  - 400 mg dose up to 1600 mg/day.

Relapse prevention—naltrexone hydrochloride is used as an aid to relapse prevention in previously dependent opiate users who have successfully completed detoxification

- It should be started at 25 mg and the dose should be increased to 50 mg/day
- The total dose may be given 3 days per week, which also aids compliance
- It is also used to facilitate *'rapid detoxification'* over 5 to 7 days in specialist centres.

Harm reduction/minimization

Harm reduction is a kind of strategy taken to reduce the morbidity and mortality for the drug users without necessarily insisting on abstinence from drugs.
A few examples include:

- Advice regarding safe sex
- Advice directed at the use of safer drugs
- Advice directed at safer routes of administration
- Advice regarding safer injecting practice
- Treatment of co-morbid mental or physical health problems
- Engagement with other sources of help
- Prescription of maintenance opiates or benzodiazepines.

Benzodiazepine detoxification

- The symptoms of benzodiazepine withdrawal appear within 24 hours of discontinuing a short-acting benzodiazepine, but may be delayed for up to 3 weeks for the longer acting benzodiazepines
- The substitute prescribing in benzodiazepine dependency uses the long-acting diazepam. Convert all benzodiazepines doses to diazepam as per Table 7.5.
- The aim is to find the lowest dose that will prevent withdrawal symptoms, and the doses should be divided to prevent over-sedation
- Cut dose by one eighth of total dose each fortnight. For low dose reduce by 2.5 mg fortnightly and for high dose reduce by 5 mg fortnightly
- Review periodically and if substantial symptoms re-emerge then the dose should be increased temporarily.

TABLE 7.5   Benzodiazepines: equivalent dosages

Drug	Dose (mg)
Diazepam	5
Lorazepam	0.5 (500 µg)
Nitrazepam	5
Temazepam	10
Chlordiazepoxide	15
Oxazepam	15

General points

- Features of alcohol withdrawal:
  - Sweating, coarse tremor, tachycardia, nausea, vomiting, generalized anxiety, psychomotor agitation, occasional visual, tactile or auditory hallucinations
  - Complicated type—5–15% by grand mal seizures

- Features of benzodiazepine withdrawals—anxiety, insomnia, headache, nausea, sweating, agitation, depersonalization, seizures, confusion and delirium
- Features of opiate withdrawal—watering eyes and nose, yawning, nausea, vomiting, diarrhoea, tremor, joint pains, muscle cramps, sweating, dilated pupils, tachycardia, hypertension, piloerection (goose-flesh)
- Features of cannabis intoxication:
  - Mild euphoria, a sense of enhanced well-being, relaxation, altered time sense, increased appetite, mild tachycardia, variable dysarthria and ataxia
  - The effects of orally smoked cannabis are slower to begin and more prolonged—if the drug is smoked, the effects of intoxication are apparent within minutes peaking in 30 minutes and lasting 2 to 5 hours
  - Acute harmful effects include mild paranoia, panic attacks and accidents
  Chronic harmful effects include anxiety, depression, dysthymia, amotivational syndrome
  - The drug is not usually associated with physical dependency but it can cause mild withdrawal symptoms including anxiety, insomnia and irritability
  - Cannabis use is associated with dose-related paranoid ideation, and can precipitate an episode or relapse of schizophrenia.

Old-age psychiatry

Old-age psychosis

The prevalence of schizophrenia (early, late and very late onset combined) in the population aged 65 years and above is believed to be about 1%.

Comparison of early-onset and late-onset (onset after 40 years of age) schizophrenia

- Similarities:
  - Genetic risk
  - Presence and severity of positive symptoms
  - Subtle brain abnormalities revealed by imaging
  - Early psychosocial maladjustments
- Differences—late onset schizophrenia has:
  - Fewer negative symptoms
  - Better response to antipsychotics
  - Better neuropsychological performance.

Characteristic features of very late-onset (after 60 years of age) schizophrenia:

- Lesser likelihood of family history of schizophrenia
- Females more affected than males
- Lesser likelihood of formal thought disorder and affective blunting
- Greater likelihood of visual hallucinations
- Associated social isolation
- Associated sensory deprivation
- Greater risk of developing tardive dyskinesia.

Psychotic symptoms of acute onset are usually seen in delirium secondary to a medical condition, drug misuse and drug-induced psychosis.

Chronic and persistent psychotic symptoms may be due to a primary psychotic disorder such as:

- Chronic schizophrenia
- Late-onset schizophrenia
- Delusional disorders
- Affective disorders
- Psychosis owing to neurodegenerative disorders, such as Alzheimer's disease, vascular dementia, dementia with Lewy bodies or Parkinson's disease
- Chronic medical conditions.

Treatment

- Antipsychotics have been the most commonly used treatment for psychotic symptoms. Their usefulness in treating schizophrenia (both late-onset and very late-onset psychosis) in elderly people is well-established
- The atypical antipsychotics, which have a better side-effect profile, are considered to be more suitable for elderly people
- More recently there have been concerns raised regarding the safety of atypical antipsychotics in psychosis due to dementia. The committee on the safety of medicine concluded that olanzapine and risperidone were associated with a two-fold increase in the risk of stroke (a small but significant risk of cerebrovascular events) in elderly patients especially in people over 80 years, and this restriction has been extended to other atypical antipsychotics
- In elderly people, age-related bodily changes affect the pharmacokinetics and pharmacodynamics of antipsychotic drugs, which have numerous side effects that can be more persistent and disabling in older people
- Follow the principle 'START LOW AND GO SLOW'

- Research literature on the use of conventional antipsychotics suggests significant improvement in psychotic symptoms with the use of haloperidol and trifluoperazine hydrochloride
- The usefulness of clozapine for treatment-resistant early-onset schizophrenia is well-established but concerns about the toxicity and the need for monitoring white cell counts due to more frequent occurrence of agranulocytosis has led to limited use in older patients and should probably be used in treatment resistance and severe tardive dyskinesia.

The recommended doses of atypical antipsychotics for elderly people are given in Table 7.6, but this should be taken as a guideline and the dosing regimen should be tailored according to the needs of individual patients.

TABLE 7.6   Recommended doses of atypical antipsychotics for elderly people

	Starting dose (mg/day)	Maximum dose (mg/day)
Olanzapine	1–5	5–15
Risperidone	0.25–0.5	2–3
Quetiapine fumrate	12.5–25	100–200
Clozapine	6.25	50–100
Ziprasidone	15–20	80–160

Psychological treatment:

- Psychological treatment involves a novel approach for older people that integrates cognitive behavioural techniques and social skills training. It aims to reduce their cognitive vulnerabilities and improve their ability to cope with stress and to adhere to other forms of treatment
- With psychosocial interventions, such as a combination of interpersonal and independent skills training together with standard occupational therapy was associated with improved social functioning and independent living.

Old-age depression

Altered symptoms in late-life depression:

- Reduced complaint of sadness
- Poor subjective memory or dementia-like picture
- Apathy and poor motivation
- Hypochondriasis and somatic concerns
- Late-onset neurotic symptoms such as late marked anxiety, obsessive-compulsive and hysterical symptoms
- Symptoms such as anorexia, weight loss and reduced energy are difficult to interpret because of co-morbid physical disorders (Koenig et al, 1997)

The most validated screening instrument is the Geriatric Depression Scale introduced in 1983.

- Depression in old age is associated with chronicity and a high risk of relapse after recovery
- Mortality is high in older patients with depression, largely because of concurrent physical disorders
- The management of depressive disorder is multimodal involving physical, psychological and social modalities, along with multidisciplinary interventions such as psychiatric nurses, social workers, occupational therapists, dieticians, speech and language therapists, physiotherapists and podiatrists.

Treatment

- The treatment for depression in people with dementia, as for depression in other older adults, includes antidepressants, psychosocial interventions or combinations of these and ECT
- For the older age group, give antidepressant treatment at an age-appropriate dose for a minimum of 6 to 8 weeks before considering that it is ineffective
- In the treatment of old-age depression, SSRIs and venlafaxine hydrochloride are to be preferred because of a favourable adverse-effects profile
- *Sertraline* has the best evidence for treatment in patients with ischaemic heart disease
- Sertraline hydrochloride and citalopram have the least potential for drug interactions
- Inappropriate antidiuretic hormone (ADH) secretion may occur as a side effect of all antidepressants, but it is more often linked with SSRIs and the risk factors include increased age, female sex and lower sodium levels
- Patients with psychotic depression usually require a combined approach with the addition of antipsychotics or ECT
- Electroconvulsive therapy remains the most effective treatment available for severe depression, particularly in psychotic depression, and the recovery rate is 80%; it is well tolerated even by very elderly people (Tew et al, 1999)
- Electroconvulsive therapy should be avoided in the first 3 months following a stroke or myocardial infarction
- Elderly patients are more likely to suffer from post-ECT confusion and cognitive impairment, which should be carefully monitored. Unilateral ECT is preferred to bilateral ECT to minimize these side effects.

Treatment-resistant depression:

- If there is a partial response within this period, treatment should be continued for a further 6 weeks as older patients take a longer time to recover, so waiting and supporting the patient may be a reasonable course of action. Consider careful monitoring for side effects and the increased risk of drug interactions

- Common augmentation strategies include lithium augmentation, combining a tricyclic with an SSRI, combinations such as SSRI and mirtazapine, high-dose venlafaxine hydrochloride.

Maintenance treatment:

- For a first episode of major depression, the patients should be kept on a continuation treatment of at least 1 year
- For patients with three or more relapses or recurrences, long-term treatment is usually recommended
- Once a patient has recovered, there is good evidence that ongoing treatment with a tricyclic, SSRI such as citalopram/sertraline hydrochloride or a combination of medication with a psychological treatment are effective
- In major depression, the combination of antidepressants with psychotherapy is more effective than either of these treatments alone, especially in relapse prevention
- Cognitive behavioural therapy is the best established psychological treatment in old-age depression, but interpersonal therapy is also effective in relapse prevention
- Family therapy has been successfully adapted for use with older adults
- Psychoeducation has been used with good effect in old-age depression.

Dementia

Investigations

Baseline blood screening tests:

- Full blood count
- Erythrocyte sedimentation rate (optional)
- Serum B12 and folate level
- Liver function tests
- Urea and electrolytes
- Thyroid function tests
- Calcium and phosphate
- Blood glucose levels
- Serum creatinine.

Further investigations:

- Mid stream urine-culture and sensitivity, urine microscopy, urine dipstick test

- Chest X-ray
- CT of the brain
- ECG
- EEG (only for specific cases)
- Lumbar puncture (only for specific cases)
- MRI of the brain (only for specific cases)
- VDRL (only for specific cases)
- HIV testing (only for specific cases)
- Screening tests such as mini mental state examination (MMSE). The MMSE is brief and simple enough for use in routine clinical practice with older patients and it is sufficiently comprehensive that when combined with other clinical measures, it provides a valuable index of dementia severity and staging.

Neuropsychological assessment—a full neuropsychological battery produces a much wider range of scores and examines more domains:

- This makes early detection of dementia possible
- It is particularly helpful in identifying dementia among people with high premorbid functioning
- It is helpful in discriminating between patients with a dementing illness and those with a focal cerebral disease.

Indications for computed tomography (CT):

- Age less than 60 years
- Sudden onset and rapid deterioration of cognitive symptoms
- Suspicion of a space-occupying lesion or normal pressure hydrocephalus
- Localized neurological signs
- Recent head trauma.

General principles of management

The management of dementia involves a broad range of key objectives including:

- Diagnosis
- Information
- Treatment of dementia
- Treatment of secondary behavioural and psychological symptoms of dementia (BPSD)
- Organization of a tailored care and support package
- Supporting carers.

The assessment should focus on three important domains:

- Diagnostic assessment
- Functional assessment
- Social assessment
- The assessment should be aimed at providing support to patients and their carers and should include a *carers' assessment* as part of it.

Medical management

- Cognitive enhancement using acetyl cholinesterase inhibitors such as donepezil hydrochloride, rivastigmine, galantamine hydrobromide and memantine hydrochloride
- Treat behavioural and psychological symptoms of dementia (BPSD) of severe intensity with antipsychotics, preferably atypical antipsychotics
- Treat depressive symptoms with antidepressants preferably SSRIs, venlafaxine hydrochloride and mirtazapine
- Treat any other medical illness and closely liaise with the geriatric team for further advice and management
- Treat insomnia with sedatives and hypnotics such as zopiclone and zolpidem tartrate.

In older people, the use of psychotropic medications is associated with a number of side effects including:

- Increased risk of falls
- Sedation/drowsiness
- Akathisia
- Parkinsonism
- Tardive dyskinesia
- Risk of cardiac arrhythmias
- Accelerated cognitive decline.

Summary of NICE guidance on acetylcholinesterases:

- Acetylcholinesterase drugs may be prescribed for patients with Alzheimer's disease with an MMSE score of 10–20 points
- Diagnosis must be made in a specialist clinic
- Assessments of cognitive functioning and activities of daily living should be made before starting drug treatment
- Only specialists should initiate treatment
- Only those likely to comply with drug treatment should be considered
- Further assessments should be made 2 to 4 months after starting treatment. If MMSE scores indicate no deterioration or improvement and there is

evidence of global or functional improvement then treatment should continue.

Acetylcholinesterases are not only useful to improve *cognitive symptoms* but research evidence has shown that they are also effective in improving the *global* outcome, improvement in *activities of daily living* (ADL) and also in controlling the *behavioural and psychological* symptoms of dementia
Common side effects of acetylcholinesterases:

- *Donepezil hydrochloride, rivastigmine, galantamine hydrobromide*— nausea, vomiting, dizziness, insomnia, diarrhoea
- *Memantine hydrochloride*—dizziness, confusion, hallucinations.

Drugs	Recommended dose
Donepezil	5–10 mg daily
Rivastigmine	1.5–6 mg BD
Galantamine	4–12 mg BD
Memantine	5–20 mg daily

Roles of other carers

Community psychiatric nurse (CPN):

- To monitor the mental state in the community, monitor compliance with medications, monitor for efficacy and tolerability of medications
- To provide additional support and can coordinate care to involve various agencies.

Occupational therapist (OT):

- To do occupational therapy assessments including home assessments—the functional assessment should focus on encouraging independence with self-care, toilet and feeding, maximizing their mobility and assisting them with communication
- To determine activities of daily living skills and level of functioning, and to ascertain the level of support needed
- To enhance their life skills training, social skills training, problem-solving skills and relaxation techniques, to regain their lost skills and to build up their confidence.

Social services:

- To help with community care assessment and assessments of needs—the social management should focus on accommodation, leisure activities,

financial matters and legal matters (power of attorney, wills) and also involved in setting up an appropriate care package including:
– Home care visits (1 to 4 per day)
– Meals-on-wheels
– Day hospital or day centre attendance
– Respite care in a residential or nursing home
– Long-term placement.

Other groups:

- *Self-help* groups
- *Support* groups
- Support through *day centres/drop-ins*
- *Supported housing*—other placements include independent flats, warden-controlled sheltered accommodation, sheltered plus accommodation, residential placement, residential EMI placement, nursing home placement
- Voluntary agencies such as the Alzheimer's Society, Age Concern and FISH
- Advocacy services.

Non-pharmacological interventions

Brief psychotherapies:

- Cognitive behavioural therapy
- Interpersonal therapy.

Most of the standard therapies and alternative therapies are usually provided in the *day hospital*.

- *Standard therapies:*
  – Behavioural therapy
  – Reminiscence therapy
  – Reality orientation
  – Validation therapy
- *Alternative therapies:*
  – Activity therapy
  – Art therapy
  – Music therapy
  – Aromatherapy
  – Bright light therapy
  – Multisensory approaches
  – Complementary therapy

- *Reminiscence therapy*—this involves helping a person with dementia to relive past experiences, especially those that might be positive and personally significant, for example, weddings, family holidays. It is seen as a way of increasing levels of well-being and providing pleasure and cognitive stimulation. It can be used with individuals or groups, and tends to use activities such as music, art and artefacts to provide stimulation
- *Reality orientation*—this therapy aims to help people with memory loss and disorientation by reminding them of facts about themselves and their environment using a range of materials and activities, such as notices, signposts and memory aids. It can be used both with individuals and with groups
- *Validation therapy*—this therapy attempts to communicate with individuals with dementia by empathizing with the feelings and meanings hidden beyond their confused speech and behaviour. As a result, the emotional content of what is being said is given more importance than the person's orientation to the present
- *Behavioural therapy*—this has been based on principles of conditioning and learning theory. It is aimed at suppressing or eliminating challenging behaviours and helps to develop more functional behaviours. It requires a detailed period of assessment to identify the ABCs (antecedents, behaviour and consequences), their relationships are made clear to the patient and the interventions are based on an analysis of these findings, changing the context in which the behaviour takes place and using reinforcement strategies that reduce the behaviour. This must be tailored to individual patients needs with a person-centred approach.

Obsessive compulsive disorder

- Depression is the most common complication of OCD, and depressive symptoms are common in OCD—as many as a third of OCD patients may fulfill the diagnostic criteria for major depression
- Many patients suffering from OCD develop co-morbid psychiatric conditions. The Co-existing diagnoses in primary OCD are major depressive disorder (65–67%), simple phobia (22%), social phobia (18%) and eating disorder.

Treatment

Most clinicians make a combined approach to the treatment of OCD that includes psychological and pharmacological treatment.

- For the successful treatment of OCD, antidepressants with potent effects on the serotonergic neurotransmitter system that appear to have anti-obsessional efficacy should be used
- OCD does not respond to antidepressants lacking 5-hydroxytryptamine (serotonin) reuptake blocking activity even though these are effective in depression
- Clomipramine has been shown to be effective in the treatment of OCD in children as well as in adults
- Random controlled trials and placebo-controlled studies have shown that fluoxetine hydrochloride, paroxetine hydrochloride, sertraline hydrochloride and fluvoxamine hydrochloride have all shown to be effective in the treatment of OCD
- The evidence supports the clinical view that higher doses of SSRIs and clomipramine than used in *depression* are likely to produce a therapeutic effect (Table 7.7)
- On the basis of risk-benefit assessment, the first choice treatment should be an SSRI. The choice should be made on the safety and tolerability, which favours SSRIs
- If treatment is initiated at lower dose then patients need to be reviewed for a possible increase in the dose if response is unsatisfactory
- Response to pharmacological treatment follows a gradual course with small increments over many months
- Most patients treated for OCD may respond within the first few weeks of treatment, but 15–20% of patients respond much later. It is, therefore, important that courses of treatment should be of adequate length
- Maintenance therapy is warranted, and higher doses may be required than standard antidepressant doses.
- Compared with clomipramine, the SSRIs have fewer side effects especially anticholinergic side effects (see below), and they have a much-improved safety profile

TABLE 7.7   Medication with demonstrated efficacy in obsessive-compulsive disorder

Drug	Dose (mg)
Clomipramine	100–300
Fluoxetine hydrochloride	30–60
Fluvoxamine hydrochloride	100–300
Paroxetine hydrochloride	40
Sertraline hydrochloride	50–200

- – Clomipramine is associated with a substantially elevated level of convulsions reported at 1.5–2% in the higher doses often used in OCD compared with 0.1–0.5% in higher doses of different SSRIs
  - – Moreover clomipramine is associated with a higher level of cardiotoxicity that is reflected in the higher rate of deaths from overdose
- Anxiolytic drugs give some short-term symptomatic relief but should not be prescribed for more than about 3 weeks at a time
- If anxiolytic treatment is needed for a longer time, small doses of an antipsychotic or tricyclic antidepressants may be used
- Long-term (up to 12 months) double-blind studies demonstrate an advantage for continuing with medication in patients who have responded to acute treatment
- There is some evidence that combination treatment is superior to psychological approaches or serotonergic antidepressant treatment when given alone.

Side effect profiles

- *Clomipramine*—sedation, orthostatic hypotension, dry mouth, blurred vision, constipation, tachycardia, urinary hesitancy or retention
- *SSRIs*—nausea, vomiting, anxiety, transient nervousness, insomnia, sexual problems, gastrointestinal disturbances.

TABLE 7.8 Treating treatment-resistant obsessive-compulsive disorder

Stage	Strategy	Treatment
1		SSRIs or clomipramine
2	Switch	SSRIs to clomipramine (vice versa)
3	Augment	Lithium, risperidone, quetiapine fumarate, trazodone hydrochloride, pindolol, haloperidol, tryptophan, buspirone hydrochloride
4	Use other treatments	Intravenous clomipramine, (rarely used) MAOIs, clonidine, clonazepam
5		Electroconvulsive therapy (rarely used)
6		Psychosurgery: cingulotomy, limbic leucotomy and anterior capsulotomy (rarely used these days)

MAOIs, monoamine oxidase inhibitors; SSRIs, selective serotonin (5-hydroxytryptamine) reuptake inhibitors

Psychological therapy

Cognitive behavioural therapy involves the cognitive part and the behavioural part:

- The cognitive part aims to identify and modify maladaptive cognitions such as perfectionist ideals, pathological doubt and magic rituals to prevent catastrophes

- The behavioural part involves exposure and response prevention and provision of alternate behaviours. Exposure techniques for obsessions, response prevention for ritualistic behaviour and thought-stopping may help in obsessional ruminations.

Obsessional rituals usually improve with a combination of exposure with response prevention to any environmental cues that increase the symptoms.

Exposure therapy:

The patient is exposed to the situations that cause anxiety or catastrophic thoughts, and this is done until the patient feels a marked relief of the anxiety symptoms. One common example for a patient with contamination fears would be to make an exposure with dirty or 'germy' objects. This provokes symptoms of anxiety and may cause severe distress for the patient, but during the course of the therapy the patient will also slowly learn from this experience that no catastrophic event will follow this exposure and so after a period of exposure for few minutes, paradoxically a decrease of anxiety symptoms occurs. This procedure has to be repeated several times with different objects that cause different levels of fear.

Response prevention:

The treatment strategy involves exposing the individual to stimuli that trigger anxiety or discomfort, and then having the individual voluntarily refrain from performing his or her ritual or compulsion. Through response-prevention techniques, the aim is to stop and prevent recurrence of the repetitive behaviour. Here again, the patient will experience anxiety and severe discomfort. But as no negative consequences occur, these negative feelings will slowly decrease, and they learn to cope with it with minimal or no anxiety. This helps the patient to face more situations that cause obsessive-compulsive behaviour.

Treatment-resistant obsessive-compulsive disorder

A treatment strategy for treatment-resistant OCD is given in Table 7.8

Anxiety disorders

Generalized anxiety disorder

If immediate management of generalized anxiety disorder (GAD) is necessary, any or all of the following should be considered (NICE, 2004)

- Support and information
- Problem-solving

- Benzodiazepines
- Sedative antihistamines
- Self-help.

Acute treatment

Pharmacological:

- Antidepressants—SSRIs such as paroxetine hydrochloride, sertraline hydrochloride and escitalopram
- Venlafaxine hydrochloride, imipramine
- Buspirone
- Benzodiazepines such as alprazolam and diazepam, which should not usually be used beyond 2 to 4 weeks

Consider an SSRI as the first-line treatment and higher doses may be associated with greater response and treatment periods of up to 12 weeks are needed to assess efficacy

For generalized anxiety disorders, the treatment is focused on predominant anxiety symptoms, but for

- Depressive symptoms—treat with antidepressants (SSRIs, TCAs, venlafaxine hydrochloride)
- Somatic symptoms—treat with benzodiazepines (lorazepam, diazepam)
- Autonomic symptoms—treat with beta blockers (atenolol, propranalol hydrochloride)
- Psychic symptoms—treat with buspirone hydrochloride.

Psychological—cognitive behavioural therapy (see below).

Long-term treatment

- Continue the drug treatment for another 6 months in patients who have shown initial response in the first 12 weeks
- If the patient responds, then continue treatment for up to a year before trial discontinuation by gradual lowering of dose
- If symptoms recur, then continue for one more year before considering a second trial discontinuation
- Treatment of co-morbid psychiatric conditions (depression, alcohol/substance misuse) is highly important and should be addressed in the early stage of treatment
- Consider cognitive behavioural therapy as it may reduce the relapse rates better than drug treatment

- If initial treatments fail, then consider combining drug treatments and cognitive behavioural therapy
- Psychosurgery should be tried if all other interventions fail for severe intractable refractory symptoms.

The interventions that have evidence for the longest duration of effect in the descending order are:

1. Psychological therapy (CBT)
2. Pharmacological therapy with antidepressants
3. Self-help.

Panic disorder (with and without agoraphobia)

A combination of pharmacological and psychological approaches is shown to be better than a single approach.

Pharmacological treatment

- *Selective serotonin reuptake inhibitors*
  - Paroxetine hydrochloride, fluoxetine hydrochloride, citalopram, sertraline hydrochloride and fluvoxamine hydrochloride have all been recommended for the treatment of panic disorders
  - Start at a low dose and increase gradually if panic symptoms increase
- *Tricyclic antidepressants*
  - TCAs such as imipramine or clomipramine have been shown to be effective
  - Other possible alternatives include amitriptyline, nortriptyline hydrochloride, desipramine, doxepin hydrochloride
- *Others*—MAOIs (e.g., phenelzine sulphate), moclobemide, venlafaxine hydrochloride and reboxetine
- *Benzodiazepines* (e.g., clonazepam, diazepam)
  - These should be used for 1 to 2 weeks in combination with antidepressants; the rationale behind this is to bring some symptomatic relief until the antidepressant becomes effective
  - They are particularly useful for severe, frequent, incapacitating symptoms. But it should be used with caution due to potential for abuse, dependence and cognitive impairment in the elderly.

If there is no significant improvement then consider switching to another evidence-based treatment after non-response at 12 weeks (change to different class of agent: SSRI, TCA, MAOI).
Psychological intervention—cognitive behavioural therapy (see below).

Longer-term treatment

Consider cognitive therapy with exposure as this may reduce relapse rates better than pharmacological treatment.

Social phobias

Pharmacological treatment

- Selective serotonin reuptake inhibitors—paroxetine hydrochloride, fluoxetine hydrochloride, citalopram, sertraline hydrochloride and fluvoxamine hydrochloride have all been recommended as first-line treatments for panic disorders
- Venlafaxine hydrochloride
- Monoamine oxidase inhibitors (e.g., phenelzine hydrochloride), moclobemide
- Anticonvulsants such as gabapentin, pregabalin
- Olanzapine
- Benzodiazepines (e.g., clonazepam)

Longer-term treatment

- Continue drug treatment for a further 6 months in patients who are responding at 12 weeks
- Consider cognitive behavioural therapy with exposure as this may reduce relapse rates better than pharmacological treatment.

Simple phobias

- Use psychological approaches based on exposure techniques as the first-line treatment
- For patients with distressing symptoms who have not responded to psychological approaches *then consider paroxetine hydrochloride or a benzodiazepine.*

Cognitive behavioural therapy for anxiety disorders

The cognitive models of anxiety disorders (generalized anxiety disorder, panic disorder, agoraphobias, social phobias) have the following in common:

- Bias in information processing
- Selective attention

- Maladaptive behaviours—safety and avoidance behaviours.

In CBT, the *cognitive* part explores the patient's automatic thoughts and beliefs in a given anxiety-provoking situation and challenges these thoughts with alternative and more plausible explanations.

It involves:

- Modification of thinking error (catastrophic misinterpretation in panic disorder, misinterpretation of any situation as threatening in GAD, misinterpretation of social threat in social phobias)
- Education about panic attacks/anxiety management
- Teaching about bodily responses associated with anxiety
- Teaching new coping skills and strategies.

The *behavioural* component involves:

- Anxiety management—use of relaxation exercises to control anxiety and control of hyperventilation
- Treating phobic avoidance by integrated exposure methods, such as modelling, graded exposure and relaxation. The *graded task assignments* break goals into achievable subtasks and help patients to achieve success step-by-step; they involve specific experiments to test negative prediction
- Behavioural experiments usually involve an exercise to induce the symptoms through imagery, role play or hyperventilation followed by asking the patient to drop their safety behaviours such as avoidance, thought control in GAD, avoidance of exercise and controlling breathing in panic disorder
- Social skills training—analysis of the skill deficits followed by teaching the skill and a period of practice within and outside the session.

Research evidence

There is strong evidence through a large number of random controlled trials for the efficacy of CBT in:

- Depression
- Agoraphobia
- Panic disorder
- Social phobia
- Specific phobia
- Obsessive-compulsive disorder
- Bulimia nervosa.

Post-traumatic stress disorder

Prevention of post-traumatic symptoms

- *De-briefing* (brief single session interventions)—routine debriefing is not indicated and should not be used in routine practice when delivering services
- *Watchful waiting*—where symptoms are mild and have been present for less than 4 weeks after the trauma, watchful waiting, as a way of managing the difficulties presented by people with PTSD, should be considered. A follow-up contact should be arranged within 1 month
- *Trauma-focused CBT* (psychological treatment) should be offered to those with severe posttraumatic symptoms lasting 1 month or longer after a traumatic event. It can prevent the emergence of chronic PTSD in individuals with post-traumatic symptoms, and it should be provided on an individual outpatient basis. The treatment should be regular and continuous, usually at least once a week, and the same person should deliver it. The duration of trauma-focused CBT should normally be 8 to 12 sessions but if initiated earlier within the first month fewer sessions may be sufficient (NICE, 2005)

Pharmacological treatment

Drug treatment should not be considered as a routine first line treatment.

Other drugs

- Selective serotonin reuptake inhibitors—*paroxetine hydrochloride*, sertraline hydrochloride, fluoxetine hydrochloride
- Tricyclic antidepressents—*amitriptyline*, imipramine
- Venlafaxine *mirtazapine*
- *Phenelzine sulphate*, lamotrigine

Higher doses of SSRIs are generally not recommended but individual patients may benefit from higher doses.

In the acute phase of PTSD for the management of sleep disturbance—use a hypnotic medication for short-term use but, if longer-term drug treatment is required, consideration should be given to the use of suitable antidepressants.

Treatment periods of up to 12 weeks are needed to assess efficacy.

Psychological treatment

Trauma-focused individual cognitive behavioural therapy

The therapist aims to explain the *traumatic event* from the patient's perspective providing *information* about the normal response to severe stress.

This involves:

- *Recall of images* of the traumatic events and *exposure* to situations that are being avoided
- *Self-monitoring* of symptoms
- *Cognitive restructuring* through the discussion of evidence for and against the patient's belief systems
- *Interpretation* of the event and attributions following the event
- *Anger management* for those who feel angry about the traumatic events and their causes
- *Anxiety management* and relaxation training.

Other psychological interventions

- Eye movement and desensitization reprocessing (EMDR)
- Supportive therapy/non-directive therapy
- Hypnotherapy
- Psychodynamic therapy.

Eye movement desensitization and reprocessing:

This is one of the new interventions used for the treatment of PTSD.

The therapist waves his or her fingers back and forth in front of the patient's eyes, and the patient is asked to track theses movements while focusing on a traumatic event. The act of tracking while concentrating seems to allow a different level of processing to occur. The patient is able to review the event more calmly or more completely than before.

It also involves a cognitive behavioural component, where the negative belief about themselves that resulted from the trauma is explored and the patient rates their level of emotions and the extent to which they believe this new belief.

Longer-term treatment

- Continue drug treatment for a further 12 months in patients who are responding at 12 weeks

- Monitor the efficacy and tolerability regularly during long-term treatment— the best evidence is for SSRIs.

Eating disorders

Anorexia nervosa

Outpatient treatment

Most people with anorexia nervosa can and should be treated in an outpatient setting. (NICE recommendations)

Outpatient management should involve a psychological treatment with physical monitoring provided by a healthcare professional competent to give it and to assess the physical risk of the illness to the patient, and the monitoring should normally continue for at least 6 months (NICE recommendations)

Inpatient treatment

Inpatient treatment should generally be reserved for situations where:

- Patients have failed to progress with appropriate outpatient therapy
- There is significant risk of suicide
- There is significant risk of severe self harm (NICE recommendations).

Patients should be admitted to a setting in which *skilled refeeding* and careful *physical monitoring* is available in combination with psychosocial interventions.

- The inpatients should follow a *structured* symptom-focused treatment regimen with the expectation of weight gain to achieve weight restoration
- The inpatients should receive psychological treatment that focuses on:
  - Eating behaviour
  - Attitudes to weight and shape and
  - On wider psychosocial issues
- In most patients with anorexia nervosa an average weekly weight gain of *0.5–1 kg* in inpatient settings and *0.5 kg* in outpatient settings should be the aim of treatment. This requires approximately *3500 to 7000* extra calories per week
- Following weight restoration, the patient should be offered outpatient psychological treatment, and typically this outpatient treatment and physical monitoring following inpatient weight restoration should continue *for at least 12 months*

- No drugs have been shown to be of specific benefit in the treatment of anorexia nervosa, therefore, the main treatment approach must be *psychological* in nature including:
  - Cognitive behavioural therapy
  - Interpersonal therapy
  - Focal psychodynamic therapy
  - Family interventions focused explicitly on eating disorders for children and adolescents (NICE recommendations)
- The therapist needs to be flexible and willing to attend to the physical as well as the psychological issues presented by the patient
- Therapists from the psychodynamic tradition may need to be *more active* than usual, but those with a cognitive behavioural approach may need to spend more time than usual exploring the complexities of their patients' attitudes to their illness
- Unfortunately, no one approach has been demonstrated to be convincingly better than the other (Fairburn, 2005)
- For adolescent patients, there is a clear consensus that it is helpful for clinicians to involve the family in treatment (Russell et al, 1987), which leads to the recommendation of conjoint family therapy involving the patient, family and therapist meeting together, or family counselling in which the clinicians meets separately with the patient and her family

A combined approach is beneficial compared with an individual approach and has a more favourable outcome.

- *Education*—nutritional education to challenge overvalued ideas, self-help manuals
- *Pharmacological*—fluoxetine hydrochloride, tricyclic antidepressants
- *Psychological*—family therapy, individual psychodynamic therapy, and cognitive behavioural therapy.

Inpatient treatment will also be considered if:

- Body mass index (BMI) is less than 13.5
- There is extremely rapid or excessive weight loss
- Severe physical health complications occur such as electrolyte imbalance, hypotension, bradycardia or hypothermia
- There is significant deterioration in mental health.

The goals of inpatient therapy should be fully discussed with the patient and the family:

- Addressing physical and psychiatric complications
- Development of a healthy meal plan

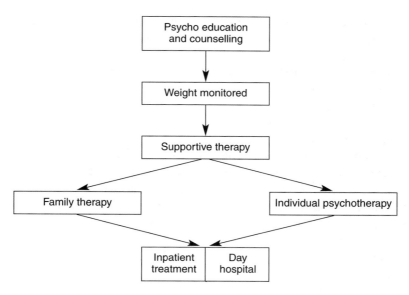

FIGURE 7.6

- Addressing underlying conflicts, such as low self-esteem and planning new coping strategies
- Enhancing communication skills (Semple et al).

Physical complications

- Endocrine changes
  - Growth hormone levels raised
  - Cortisol (positive DST) level raised
  - Gonadotrophin levels decreased
  - Oestrogen level decreased
  - Testosterone level decrease
  - T3 levels decreased
  - Amenorrhoea/loss of libido
- Metabolic abnormalities
  - Dehydration, hypoglycemia and impaired glucose tolerance, hyper-cholesterolaemia
  - Deranged liver function tests, hypokalemia, hypoproteinemia
  - Plasma amylase (raised), lowered calcium, magnesium and phosphate levels
- Haematological problems
  - Normochromic, normocytic or iron-deficient anaemia

- Leucopenia, with a relative lymphocytosis, low erythrocyte sedimentation rate (ESR), hypocellular marrow
- Cardiovascular problems
  - Peripheral oedema, congestive cardiac failure, bradycardia, hypotension
  - Decreased heart size, QT prolongation
- Gastrointestinal problems
  - Swollen salivary glands, dental caries, erosion of enamel (vomiting)
  - Delayed gastric emptying, acute gastric dilations (bulimic episodes, vigorous refeeding, constipation), acute pancreatitis
- Renal problems
  - Acute/chronic renal failure, hypokalemic nephropathy
  - Proteinuria and reduced glomerular filtration rate (GFR), raised urea and creatinine
- Musculoskeletal problems
  - Osteoporosis, pathological myopathy, proximal myopathy, stunted growth
  - Muscle cramps.

Bulimia nervosa

Primary care—self-help programme

Six steps in self-help manual:

1. Monitoring
2. Establishing a meal plan
3. Learning to intervene
4. Problem-solving
5. Eliminating dieting
6. Changing your mind.

Combined approaches improve outcomes.

Outpatient treatment

- Antidepressant treatment—SSRIs (especially fluoxetine hydrochloride at a higher dose of 60 mg) are the drugs of first choice for the treatment of bulimia nervosa in terms of acceptability, tolerability and reduction of symptoms. Long-term treatment for more than 1 year is usually necessary
- Group therapy—guided self-help (bibliotherapy) is useful with education and support, often in a group setting. The treatment usually takes about 4 months and requires 8–10 meetings with the facilitator, appropriate for patients in primary care settings.

Specialist unit

Individual therapy:

- Inpatient care—recommended in the following situations:
  - If the patient is at high risk of suicide or severe self-harm
  - There are severe physical health problems
  - In refractory cases
  - If the patient is pregnant and the risk of abortion is high
- Cognitive behavioural therapy—course of treatment should be for 16 to 20 sessions over 4 to 5 months. CBT, the preferred psychotherapeutic treatment for bulimia nervosa aims to normalize eating habits and congnitive techniques are designed to modify the excessive concerns about shape and weight. CBT is also helpful to bring improvement in mood symptoms, social functioning and self-esteem also improve with well-maintained effects and low relapse rates
- Interpersonal psychotherapy—may be effective in the long-term but acts less quickly.

Specific physical health problems associated with bulimia nervosa

- Electrolyte disturbances—hyponatraemia, hypokalemia
- Vomiting—metabolic alkalosis
- Dental erosion
- Constipation
- Oesophageal erosions
- Gastric and duodenal ulcers
- Pancreatitis
- Leucopenia and lymphocytosis
- Arrhythmias and cardiac failure.

8

Prognosis

- The examiners usually explore the prognostic factors for each particular case
- You are expected to review the favourable and poor prognostic factors, both in terms of the immediate outcome concerning the particular episode and the longer-term
  - In this context, the candidate can present the immediate prognosis as good but draw attention to the poorer long-term prognosis.
- Any statements that you make must be justifiable and it may lead to further questioning by the examiner.

Consider:

- Immediate/short term – good and poor prognostic factors
- Long term – good and poor prognostic factors.

Schizophrenia

Good prognostic factors

- Acute or abrupt onset
- Late onset of the illness
- Short duration
- Presence of precipitating stressor
- Female sex
- First episode of the illness
- Presence of family history of mood disorder
- Good social support
- No history of co-morbid substance misuse

- Good premorbid personality traits
- Presence of mood symptoms
- Presence of positive symptoms
- Presence of good insight
- Good compliance with treatment

Poor prognostic factors

- Insidious onset
- Early age of onset
- Chronic course of the illness
- Absence of precipitating stressor
- Male sex
- Past history of similar episodes
- Family history of schizophrenia
- Poor social support
- Co-morbid substance misuse
- Poor premorbid adjustment
- Absence of mood symptoms
- Presence of negative symptoms
- Lack of insight
- Poor compliance with treatment
- Institutionalization or long-term hospitalization.
- Low premorbid IQ
- The longer the duration of untreated illness.

Best predictors of relapse in the short term

- Non-compliance with medications
- High expressed emotion
- Stressful life events (3 weeks prior to relapse).

Schizoaffective disorder

Depressive symptoms are more likely to run a chronic course compared with manic presentation. The good/poor prognostic factors are the same as those for schizophrenia.

Mood disorders

Good prognostic factors

- Acute or abrupt onset
- Earlier age of onset
- Typical clinical features
- Severe depression
- Well-adjusted premorbid personality
- Good response to treatment.

Poor prognostic factors

- Insidious onset
- Later age of onset (elderly patient)
- Time to initial treatment
- Long duration of index episode
- Severe index episode
- High number of previous episodes
- Family history of affective disorder
- Recent major stressful life events
- Co-morbid anxiety
- Co-morbid substance misuse
- Co-morbid physical disease
- Co-morbid personality disorders
- Premorbid neuroticism
- Underlying dysthymia
- Unfavourable early environment
- Mood-incongruent psychotic features
- Poor drug compliance
- Marked hypochondriacal features
- Double depression.

Clues to possible bipolarity for patients with unipolar depression

- Early age of onset
- Recurrent episodes of depression, usually of short duration
- History of bipolar disorders in relatives
- Presence of psychotic features

- Post partum onset
- Poor or short-lived response to antidepressants
- Manic symptoms induced by antidepressants or electroconvulsive therapy
- Atypical depressive features, such as weight gain or hyperphagia.

The prognosis for bipolar disorder is worse than for unipolar disorder, both in terms of recurrences and recovery. When compared to unipolar disorders, the bipolars showed more frequent but shorter episodes. Late onset of affective illness was associated with chronicity and recovery was more frequent among unipolar than among bipolar patients.

Follow-up studies over 25 years show a definite recovery in:

- 25% of depressed patients
- 16% of bipolar patients.

Drug and alcohol misuse

Good prognostic factors

- Patient motivated to change
- Patient accepting of appropriate treatment goal
- Supportive family or relationships
- Patient in employment
- 'Alcoholics Anonymous' (AA) involvement
- Treatable co-morbid illness, such as social phobia or anxiety.

Poor prognostic factors

- Ambivalent to change
- Homelessness
- Unstable accommodation
- Repeated treatment failures
- Cognitive impairment
- Drinking embedded into lifestyle.

Obsessive-compulsive disorder

Good prognostic factors

- Good premorbid social and occupational functioning

- Clear precipitating event
- Episodic symptoms.

Poor prognostic factors

- Early onset
- Longer duration of illness
- Co-morbid depression
- Bizarre compulsions
- Giving in to compulsions
- Overvalued ideas or delusional beliefs
- History of personality disorder (schizotypal PD).

Eating disorders

Anorexia nervosa

Good prognostic factors

- Younger age of onset
- No bulimic episodes
- Less number of previous hospitalizations

Poor prognostic factors

- Male sex
- Late age of onset
- Duration of the illness (chronic)
- Excessive weight loss
- Bulimic features (vomiting/purging)
- Poor parental relationships
- Poor childhood maladjustments/premorbid personality traits
- Anxiety when eating with others
- Poor social support
- Extreme treatment avoidance—compulsory treatment required.

Bulimia nervosa

Poor prognostic factors

- Severe personality disorder
- Low self-esteem.

Alzheimer's dementia

Poor prognostic factors

- Male sex
- Onset before 65 years of age
- Prominent behavioural problems
- Presence of mood symptoms, such as depression
- Parietal lobe damage
- Severe focal cognitive deficits, such as apraxia
- Absence of misidentification syndromes.

9

Miscellaneous topics

Suicide

Static and stable risk factors

- Age—older age
- Sex—male
- Marital status
- Childhood adversity
- Family history of suicide
- History of mental disorder
- Previous hospitalization
- History of substance use disorder
- Personality disorder/traits—impulsive or aggressive.

Dynamic risk factors

- Active psychological symptoms
- Active suicidal ideation, communication and intent
- Feelings of guilt, hopelessness, worthlessness and depressive features
- Treatment adherence
- Psychosocial stressors
- Alcohol and substance misuse
- Psychiatric admission and discharge
- Social support—housing, employment, financial status, family support.

Future risk factors for suicide

- Access to preferred methods of suicide
- Future stressors in life

- Future service contact
- Future response to drug treatment
- Future response to psychosocial intervention.

Deliberate self-harm

Risk factors

- Sex—female
- Age—younger age of onset
- Divorced, single, widowed, married
- Lower social class
- Unemployed
- Personality disorder
- Substance misuse.

Risk factors for repetition of self-harm

- Previous history of self-harm
- Alcohol and drug abuse
- Criminal record and history of violence
- Personality disorder—antisocial personality
- Psychiatric treatment
- Unemployment
- Lower social class
- High suicidal intent
- Hopelessness
- Non-compliance with treatment.

The association between suicide and mental illness is given in Table 9.1.

TABLE 9.1 Association between suicide and mental illness

Illness	Percentage of people with this illness who commit suicide	Percentage of people who commit suicide who have this illness
Schizophrenia	10	5
Depression	15	70
Alcoholism	15	15

Drug prescribing for specialist populations

Psychotropic prescribing in pregnancy

- Antipsychotics—low-dose chlorpromazine, low-dose haloperidol, low-dose trifluoperazine hydrochloride
- Antidepressants—fluoxetine hydrochloride, amitriptyline, imipramine, nortriptyline
- Anxiolytics and hypnotics—benzodiazepines are best avoided, but for sedation promethazine is widely used
- Mood stabilizers—better to avoid unless risks and consequences of relapse outweigh known risk of teratogenesis
- Lithium
  - Increased risk of Ebstein's anomaly (1:1000)
  - However, the relapse rates are quite high—50% within 1–2 months on discontinuation is regarded to preclude stopping lithium therapy in pregnancy
  - Detailed ultrasound or foetal echocardiography is indicated at 16–18 weeks
  - Serum monitoring, dosage adjustment, particularly during the second and third trimesters; also ensuring adequate hydration after delivery is important
- Sodium valproate and carbamazepine
  - Sodium valproate and carbamazepine are associated with neural tube defects
  - Detailed ultrasonography should be carried out at 16–18 weeks
  - Maternal serum alpha protein levels should be measured at 16–18 weeks
  - Folic acid supplementation is recommended for women of childbearing age
  - Vitamin K should be given to mothers in the last month of pregnancy and to neonates at birth due to the risk of neonatal haemorrhage.

Psychotropic prescribing in lactation

- Antipsychotics—sulpiride, olanzapine
- Antidepressants—sertraline hydrochloride, paroxetine hydrochloride, imipramine, nortriptyline hydrochloride
- Mood stabilizers—to be avoided if possible; lithium should be avoided; carbamazepine and sodium valproate should be used cautiously, to be given as a single dose in slow-release form
- Anxiolytics and hypnotics—lorazepam, zolpidem tartrate.

Psychotropic prescribing for patients with renal impairment

No drug is clearly preferred to another. They should be used with caution in exceptional circumstances.

- Antipsychotics—low dose haloperidol (2–5 mg/day), low dose olanzapine (5 mg /day)
- Antidepressants—sertraline hydrochloride, citalopram
- Mood stabilizers—sodium valproate, carbamazepine, lamotrigine at lower doses
- Anxiolytics and hypnotics—lorazepam, zopiclone.

Psychotropic prescribing for patients with hepatic impairment

- Antipsychotics—low dose haloperidol (2–5 mg/day), sulpiride, amisulpride, low doses of atypical agents
- Antidepressants—low dose: imipramine, paroxetine hydrochloride, citalopram
- Mood stabilizers—lithium, gabapentin
- Anxiolytics and hypnotics—lorazepam, temazepam, oxazepam, zopiclone.

Psychotropic prescribing for patients with cardiovascular disease

Post-myocardial infarction patients:

- Antidepressants—selective serotonin (5-hydroxytryptamine) reuptake inhibitors (SSRIs), such as fluoxetine hydrochloride, paroxetine hydrochloride, sertraline hydrochloride, and low-dose trazadone
- Antipsychotics—low-dose haloperidol, olanzapine
- Avoid phenothiazines, tricyclic antidepressants, beta-blockers, and hypotensive agents such as clozapine, risperidone, and high-dose venlafaxine hydrochloride.

Psychotropic prescribing for patients with epilepsy

- Antipsychotics—haloperidol, sulpiride, amisulpride, zuclopenthixol, risperidone, quetiapine fumarate
- Antidepressants—SSRIs
- Mood stabilizers—carbamazepine, sodium valproate, lamotrigine, therapeutic doses of lithium
- Anxiolytics and hypnotics—all benzodiazepines can be used, as they are anticonvulsant in nature.

Psychotropic prescribing for patients with post-stroke depression

- SSRIs
- Nortriptyline hydrochloride.

Monitoring

Recommended plasma levels for selected drugs are given in Table 9.2.

TABLE 9.2   Recommended plasma levels for selected drugs

Drug	Recommended plasma level
Nortriptyline hydrochloride	50–150 µg/L
Amitriptyline	100–200 µg/L
Clozapine	350–500 µg/L
Olanzapine	20–40 µg/L
Lithium	0.8–1.2 mmol/L
Carbamazepine	4–12 mg/L
Sodium valproate	50–125 mg/L
Phenytoin	10–20 mg/L

Recommended monitoring for newer antipsychotics

- Baseline:
  - Full blood count
  - Urea and electrolytes
  - Blood lipids
  - Liver function tests
  - Glycosylated haemoglobin
  - Weight
  - Blood pressure
  - Electrocardiogram (ECG; optional)
- Glycosylated haemoglobin, urea and electrolytes, liver function tests should be repeated after 6 months and then yearly
- Creatinine phosphokinase if neuroleptic malignant syndrome is suspected
- Electrocardiogram when maintenance dose is reached
- Electroencephalogram, if myoclonus or seizures occur
- Prolactin level, if symptoms of hyperprolactinemia occur
- Blood lipids—after 3 months and then yearly.

Recommended monitoring for Clozapine

- Perform baseline blood tests (white cell count and differential count) before starting clozapine
- Full blood count—weekly for the first 18 weeks, then at least every 2 weeks for 1 year and monthly thereafter.
- Daily monitoring of pulse, temperature and blood pressure for at least the first 2 weeks after initiating the treatment.

Additional monitoring requirements

- Baseline—weight, glycosylated haemoglobin, liver function tests
- One month—weight, plasma glucose
- Three months—weight, glycosylated haemoglobin
- Six months—weight, glycosylated haemoglobin, liver function tests
- Twelve months—weight, glycosylated haemoglobin.

Consider also use of ECG where available and also monitor plasma lipids.

Recommended monitoring for lithium

Pre-lithium work up: FBC, liver function tests, renal function tests, thyroid function tests, ECG, urea and electrolytes.

- Start at 400 mg once daily
- Plasma level
  - Check after 5 to 7 days
  - Then check every 5 to 7 days until the required therapeutic level is reached
  - Once stable, check every 3 to 6 months
- Check thyroid function and kidney function tests every 6 months.

Recommended monitoring for carbamazepine

- Perform full blood count at baseline and every 2 weeks for the first 2 months and then every 3 to 6 months
- Monitor serum carbamazepine levels every 2 weeks for first 2 months and then every 3 to 6 months.

Recommended monitoring for sodium valproate

- Perform full blood count at baseline and then 6 monthly
- Check hepatic and renal function at baseline and then 6 monthly.

Anticholinergic medication

Side effects—dryness of the mouth, constipation, urinary hesitancy, blurred vision, dilation of the pupils, tachycardia, dizziness, euphoria, hallucinations, delirium.

Recommended doses are given in Table 9.3.

TABLE 9.3   Recommended doses for anti-cholinergic drugs

Drug name	Usual recommended dosage (mg/day)
Procyclidine hydrochloride	2.5–30
Orphenadrine	150–400
Benztropine mesilate	0.5–6
Benzhexol hydrochloride	2–15

Benzodiazepines

Side effects—drowsiness, dizziness, ataxia, respiratory depression, disinhibition in the elderly.

Recommended doses are given in Table 9.4.

TABLE 9.4   Recommended doses for benzodiazepines

Drug name	Recommended dosages (mg/day)
Lorazepam	1–4
Temazepam	10–20
Nitrazepam	5–10
Oxazepam	15–90
Diazepam	2–30
Chlordiazepoxide	10–100
Alprazolam	0.25–1.5

Non-benzodiazepine alternatives

Side effects:

- Zopiclone—bitter taste, sedation, dry mouth, headaches, fatigue
- Zolpidem tartrate—headache, dizziness, drowsiness, gastrointestinal upsets
- Buspirone hydrochloride—headaches, drowsiness, dizziness, nausea.

Recommended doses are given in Table 9.5.

TABLE 9.5   Recommended doses for non-benzodiazepine alternatives

Drug name	Recommended dosages (mg/day)
Zopiclone	7.5–1.5
Zolpidem tartrate	5–10
Buspirone hydrochloride	10–45

Neuropsychometric assessment

The patient will be asked to answer sets of questions to assess their overall intellectual and cognitive function, normalized to the patient's age and baseline and educational level.

The standard neuropsychometric testing battery has the following components:

- Attention
- Abstraction and problem-solving
- Memory
- Orientation
- Motor
- Verbal
- Perceptual/constructional
- Estimated premorbid verbal IQ
- Depression.

These tests should be performed for any patient that the clinician suspects to have cognitive impairment and/or dementia.

Self-help

- Discuss with the patient about what they can do to help themselves. For example:
  - Adhere to treatment plan and take their medications
  - Avoid precipitating factors, such as drug and alcohol misuse
  - Consider modification of lifestyle—do physical activity, consume a healthy diet, avoid smoking etc.
- Provide written self-help manuals and leaflets appropriate to the current disorder
- Encourage attendance at self-help groups, voluntary treatment organizations and patient organizations.

Good luck and all the best.

Drugs list

alprazolam
amisulpride
amoxapine
antabuse (disulfiram)
aripiprazole
atenolol
biperiden
buprenorphine
carbamazepine
chlordiazepoxide
chlorpromazine
cimetidine
citalopram
clomipramine
clonazepam
clozapine
desipramine
dexamethasone
diazepam
disulfiram
escitalopram
flupenthixol decanoate
fluphenazine decanoate
gabapentin
glycine
haloperidol
haloperidol decanoate
ibuprofen

imipramine
isocarboxazid
isoniazid,
lamotrigine
levodopa,
lorazepam
methyldopa,
mirtazapine,
moclobemide
nitrazepam
olanzapine
orlistat
orphenadrine
oxazepam
phenytoin
pindolol
pregabalin
promethazine
reboxetine
reserpine,
risperidone
rivastigmine
sibutramine
sodium valproate
sulpiride
temazepam
topiramate
trimipramine

tryptophan
ziprasidone
zopiclone
zotepine

zuclopenthixol
zuclopenthixol acetate
zuclopenthixol decanoate

Drug name changes to rINN

acamprosate	acamprosate calcium
amitryptyline	amitriptyline
D-amphetamine	amphetamine
benzhexol	benzhexol hydrochloride
benztrophine	benzatropine mesilate
bromocriptine	bromocriptine mesilate
buspirone	buspirone hydrochloride
clonidine	clonidine hydrochloride
D-cycloserine	cycloserine
cyclosporine	ciclosporin
cyproheptadine	cyproheptadine hydrochloride
donepezil	donepezil hydrochloride
L-dopa,	levodopa
dothiepin	dothiepin hydrochloride
doxepin	doxepin hydrochloride
duloxetine	duloxetine hydrochloride
fluoxetine	fluoxetine hydrochloride
flupenthixol	flupenthixol decanoate
fluvoxamine	fluvoxamine malate
galantamine	galantamine hydrobromide
levothyroxine	thyroxine sodium
lofepramine	lofepramine hydrochloride
Lofexidine	Lofexidine hydrochloride
loperamide	loperamide hydrochloride
maprotiline	maprotiline hydrochloride
memantine	memantine hydrochloride
methadone	methadone hydrochloride
methyl phenidate	methyl phenidate hydrochloride
metoclopramide	metoclopramide hydrochloride
mianserin	mianserin hydrochloride
naltrexone	naltrexone hydrochloride
nefazodone	nefazodone hydrochloride
nortryptyline	nortriptyline hydrochloride

paroxetine	paroxetine hydrochloride
phenelzine	phenelzine sulfate
pipothiazine decanoate	pipotiazine decanoate
procyclidine	procyclidine hydrochloride
propranolol	propranolol hydrochloride
quetiapine	quetiapine fumarate
sertraline	sertraline hydrochloride
sildenafil	sildenafil citrate
tranylcypromine	tranylcypromine sulfate
trazodone	trazodone hydrochloride
trifluoperazine	trifluoperazine hydrochloride
trihexyphenidyl	trihexyphenidyl hydrochloride
triiodothyronine	liothyronine sodium
venlafaxine	venlafaxine hydrochloride
vincristine	vincristine sulfate
yohimbine	yohimbine hydrochloride
zolpidem	zolpidem tartrate

References and further reading

References

Barbui C, Campomori A, D'Avanzo B, Negri E, Garattini S. (1999) Antidepressant drug use in Italy since the introduction of SSRIs: national trends, regional differences and impact on suicide rates. *Soc Psychiatry Psychiatr Epidemiol* **34**:152–6.

Chick J, Ritson B, Connaughton J, Stewart A, Chick J. (1988) Advice versus extended treatment for alcoholism: a controlled study. *Br J Addict* **83**:159–70.

Edwards G, Gross MM. (1976) Alcohol dependence: provisional description of a clinical syndrome. *Br Med J* **1**:1058–61.

Edwards G, Guthrie S. (1967) A controlled trial of inpatient and outpatient treatment of alcohol dependency. *Lancet* **1**:555–9.

Fairburn CG. (2005) Evidence-based treatment of anorexia nervosa. *Int J Eat Disord* **37** Suppl:S26–30; discussion S41–2.

Folstein MF, Folstein SE, McHugh PR. (1975) Mini-mental state. A practical method for grading the cognitive state of patients for the clinician. *J Psychiatr Res* **12**:189–98.

Koenig HG, George LK, Peterson BL, Pieper CF. (1997) Depression in medically ill hospitalized older adults: prevalence, characteristics, and course of symptoms according to six diagnostic schemes. *Am J Psychiatry* **154**:1376–83.

Lieberman JA, Koreen AR, Chakos M et al. (1996) Factors influencing treatment response and outcome of first-episode schizophrenia: implications for understanding the pathophysiology of schizophrenia. *J Clin Psychiatry* **57** Suppl 9:5–9.

McGrath J, Saha S, Welham J, El Saadi O, MacCauley C, Chant D. (2004) A systematic review of the incidence of schizophrenia: the distribution of rates and the influence of sex, urbanicity, migrant status and methodology. *BMC Med* **2**:13.

Miller WR, Hester RK. (1986) Inpatient alcoholism treatment. Who benefits? *Am Psychol* **41**:794–805.

Pane FJ, Ringer L, Ferguson L, Koshko N. (1991) Notifying patients of adverse drug reactions. *Am J Hosp Pharm* **48**:236–7.

Robinson DG, Woerner MG, Alvir JM et al. (1999) Predictors of treatment response from a first episode of schizophrenia or schizoaffective disorder. *Am J Psychiatry* **156**:544–9.

Russell GF, Szmukler GI, Dare C, Eisler I. (1987) An evaluation of family therapy in anorexia nervosa and bulimia nervosa. *Arch Gen Psychiatry* **44**:1047–56.

Semple D, Smyth R, Burns J, Darjee R, McIntosh A. (2005) Oxford Handbook of Psychiatry. OUP, Oxford.

Strang J, Marsden J, Cummins M et al. (2000) Randomized trial of supervised injectable versus oral methadone maintenance: report of feasibility and 6–month outcome. *Addiction* **95**:1631–45.

Tew JD Jr, Mulsant BH, Haskett RF et al. (1999) Acute efficacy of ECT in the treatment of major depression in the old. *Am J Psychiatry* **156**:1865–70

Further reading

Ahuja N. (2001) *A Short Texbook of Psychiatry*. 4E, Jaypee Brothers Medical Publishers Ltd., London.

Andrews G, Jenkins R. (1999) *Management of Mental Disorders* 2E. WHO Collaborating Centers for Mental Health and Substance Abuse. Geneva.

British National Formulary, No 50. (2005) BMJ Publishing, London.

Gelder M, Cowen P, Harrison P. (2006) 5E *Shorter Oxford Textbook of Psychiatry*, OUP, Oxford.

Goodwin G, Sachs G. (2004) *Bipolar Affective Disorder*. Icon Group International.

ICD-10 Classification of Mental Behavioral Disorders, Clinical Descriptions and Diagnostic Guidelines 2E. (2002) AITBS Publishers and Distributors.

Kane JM. (2000) *Management issues in schizophrenia*. 1E, Martin Dunitz, Abington.

Lewis SW, Buchanan RW. (2002) *Schizophrenia*: Fast Facts in Psychiatry. 2E. Fine Print Services Ltd. Oxford.

Murthy SPM (2004) *Get Through MRCPsych part 1*. RSM Press, London.

Semple D, Smyth R, Burns J, Darjee R, McIntosh A. (2005) Oxford Handbook of Psychiatry. OUP, Oxford.

Taylor D, Paton C, Kerwin R.(2005–06) The Maudsley Prescribing Guidelines, 8E, Cromwell Press Ltd, Trowbridge, Wilts.

Williams C, Trigwell P, Yeomans D. (2002) Pass the MRCPsych Part 1 and 2 2E, WB Saunders, London.

NICE guidelines

British Association of psychopharmacology guidelines
Bipolar affective disorder—Guy Goodwin and Gary Sachs
Advances in psychiatric treatment Jan 2004–Jan 2006
A short textbook of psychiatry—Niraj Ahuja